Verity Red

PART THREE

Verity Red

PART THREE

Maria de la Mann

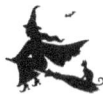

easyBroom

Verity Red

PART THREE

An easyBroom book

Copyright © 2020 Maria de la Mann

ISBN 978-0957628854

Illustrations and Cover Design: Maria de la Mann

A catalogue record of this book is available from
The British Library

Books by the author

Verity Red's Diary (*A story of surviving M.E.*)

Love & Best Witches

Verity Writes Again

Verity Red (part one)

Verity Red (part two)

for Shauna, Sarah, and Sally

Dedicated to the memory of

Cleopatra, Purrdita and Tinkerbell

Acknowledgements

I always thank my cats last. So this time I will thank them first. For their warm, furry company while I wrote and illustrated this book, endless inspiration, and treading nicely on my laptop keys to improve my writing.

A whole trilogy of thankyous to my partner Nigel for his time and patience, helping me put together *another* book. And to his dear sister Julia, for doing another *most agreeable* job, proof reading this final book of my trilogy.

Last, but not least, many thanks to my favourite poet, Jim Logan, for his lovely poem about seashells.

Prologue

Verity Red feels she has suddenly aged – and wonders *why?*

What is in the large unexpected parcel?

Is her next appointment going to be *another* disaster?

Why does she text Ben to say she has been a naughty girl?

What happened at the seaside?

Why is Verity outside a stranger's house, peering through the window?

What happens next?

Read on....

June

Sunday 1ˢᵗ

8.30 a.m.   I'm staring at my face in bathroom mirror..... UGH! Extra pale. Dragged-through-the-forest hair. Eyes like two mouldy blueberries, half-sunken in a bowl of cold porridge. And I look fifty years older than I did yesterday morning. WHY?

8.31 a.m.   How did that happen? Why *fifty years older?*......... Hmm...... Most probably because I overdid it at the Faerie Festival – *a lot!*

8.32 a.m.   *And* when I smiled in the mirror yesterday, I would have looked my best. *I was* wearing lovely fairy make-up: woodland-green eyeshadows, lashings of mascara, concealer under my eyes, wild rose blusher on my cheeks. Pixie-pink lipstick.

8.33 a.m.   I'm sitting on side of bath... sighing.... and yawning. I'm bound to look a little weathered after frolicking in a wild woodland clearing with fairy folk, close to the windy Sussex coastline.

8.36 a.m.   Still sitting on side of bath, deep in thought – instead of sitting in a nice deep bath (no energy for that). Last week, when I mentioned to Ben that some vegetables needed eating up before they went soft and wrinkly, he said, 'Like you!'

8.37 a.m.   Today I feel (and must look like) an old vegetable. Or a fruit – my mascara smudged eyes are the bruised bits. But was it *really* worth it?

8.38 a.m.   ***YES! YES! YES!***

8.37 a.m.   I may not be in the bath, but I'm splashing about in beautiful bubbles of memories. They keep popping into my mind.

8.38 a.m.   POP! POP! POP! Wonderful.

* * * * * * * *

9.15 a.m.   Purrdita is playing inside an old carrier bag. She sticks her head out through one of the handles, twitching her whiskers. Ben walks into the room and laughs.

ME: One of the many reasons cats are so great, is they find a wrinkly old bag, fun and fascinating.

BEN: You are still fun and fascinating dear.

ME: That's sweet of you to say.

BEN: On a good day.

* * * * * * * *

2.20 p.m.   Ben sits next to me on the garden bench. We watch a tiny blue butterfly flutter by.

ME: Time *really flew* yesterday.

BEN: Like the people dancing and fluttering around in fairy costumes. I can't remember when I last saw you enjoy yourself so much.

ME: Mmm, yes..... this is delicious by the way.

BEN: Very tasty.

ME: And light (crumby smile).

BEN: Delicate flavour.

ME: Light and delicate, like a fairy cake should be. And they're *real* fairy cakes, because we bought them at a Faerie Festival. They make my eyelashes flutter (fluttering eyelashes).

BEN: Like that blue butterfly above your head.

ME: Maybe it's a bluebell fairy spirit.

BEN: Yes dear (brushing crumbs off his belly).

ME: That must have been a strawberry fairy on my cake, the little pink icing fairy was strawberry flavour. What fairy did you have?

BEN: A yellow, *lemon fairy* (feigns sheer delight).

ME: The buttercups look like little cups of sunshine dancing in the breeze, between the blades of grass, don't they!....... Miniature yellow cups on Mother Nature's fresh green tablecloth.

BEN: When it rains, does she wash them in *mild green* fairy liquid?

ME: Of course.

BEN: Do you feel a poem coming on?

ME: No. Not today.

BEN: You were like a buttercup, doing a little wiggle between tall, thin, green pixies at the festival.

ME: I can barely move today. Don't know where I got the energy. Must have been the fairy mead, fabulous music, and freshly made pizza with a fairy ring of mushrooms on top......... I'm *so very glad* you're on holiday now (big sigh, shoulders and eyelids drooping, head flopping to one side).

BEN: Do you fancy a cuppa?

ME: Ooh, *yes please!*

* * * * * * * * *

2.36 p.m. We sip minty tea. Our thoughts, miles away with the fairies again.

ME: The Celtic psy-folk band were very good.

BEN: Flutatious. Yes excellent, especially the flautist and fiddle player.

ME: Pixiephonic were fun. The singer looked like a pixie too, especially with his prosthetic pointy ears.

BEN: How do you know they were prosthetic?

ME: *He, he......* I loved the acoustic folk songs, with tales of witches, fairies and magic......... *Oooh!* (rubbing shoulder) I think I'm going to have serious wing-flop for a few weeks. Or months.

BEN: Was it worth it?

ME: Definitely! I'm looking forward to going next year. I'd love to go on a day when the Roving Crows are playing.

BEN: We're going next year?

ME: Oh yes. Even if my wings have dropped off.

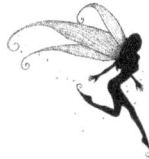

Monday 2nd

11.20 a.m.   Ben plods in through the front door, laden with orange Sainsbury's carrier bags, carries them through to the kitchen, then begins to unpack. Bored after Saturday's excitement, I watch this lively entertainment.

ME: This looks lovely – Fairy Tomato and Lime soup!

BEN: Erm, it's....

ME: Sounds tasty. It's seasoned with garlic, ginger, black pepper and witchy coriander. You'll like it because it's got red chillies too, good for your diet.

BEN: You've got your M.E. eyeballs in today, look at the front of the carton again.

ME: Oh. *Fiery* Tomato and Lime soup. We can pretend it's a fairy soup...... Maybe I'll suggest Covent Garden soups do a fairy ring mushroom soup. They did a good one for Halloween last year, remember?

BEN: Yeah, Witches' Brew.

ME: With blood red plum tomatoes.

BEN: And eyeballs.

ME: Eyeballs?!

BEN: Black eyed peas.

ME: Oh yes. It was very low calorie too, perfect for your diet. And Halloween being the end of a month, it was your weigh day. And that reminds me, we forgot it was weigh day on Saturday, we were too busy....

BEN: Flying off to fairyland. I'm not bothered we forgot, I was a naughty boy last month.

ME: Never mind, we'll wait till the end of this month.

BEN: Ah. I'm on holiday, I –

ME: Will be indulging in big, fat, hot chips at the seaside, with me or Bill........ meals with mates or family......... vegetable massala.... onion bhaji.... sag aloo.

BEN: I really fancy an Indian now. Or Chinese.

ME: Mmm...... mushroom chop suey...... bean sprouts.... fried bamboo shoots and water chestnuts..... sweet and....

BEN: Sour veg. Shall we treat ourselves to Chinese tonight?

ME: Why not! Oh, I like these purple carrots, I've never seen them before (holding one on the end of my nose and cackling). But I can't eat them at the moment.

BEN: Why not?

ME: They're a root vegetable. Wanda of Weekly Witch says they are grounding, like beetroot. But I don't want to feel grounded yet, I want to feel up in the air, away with the fairies. Well, for a few more days anyway.

BEN: Anything you say dear.

* * * * * * * * *

2.20 p.m. I'm in the garden, tying my purchase from the festival to the bird table. And as I watch it twirl, Ben joins me (brushing fairy cake crumbs off his cheek).

ME: Isn't she *beautiful!*

BEN: Delightful. Cleverly sculpted wire.

ME: I couldn't resist her. She's a miniature version of the huge sculptures of fairy folk at Trentham Gardens in Staffordshire, by Robin Wight. I saw some of his work advertised in Weekly Witch years ago, I'd love to visit the gardens one day.

BEN: We will.

ME: For now I'll enjoy my tiny version. I like the way the sun sparkles on her mesh wings and long, copper hair. She looks quite at home already. I'm sure the seven dwarves, pixie and fairy garden ornaments will approve!

BEN: I expect you were tempted to buy most of what was on the craft stalls.

ME: That's a big, fat, YES! (eyes glowing – miles away). The ornamental dragons, unicorns, pixies, black cats and witches....

BEN: Cauldrons, candles and crystals.

ME: Spell books, fairytale jewellery, sun catchers.

BEN: Floaty fairy frocks.

ME: In pastel or woodland-green shades (far away in fairy-land look).

BEN: You were most restrained dear.

ME: I could see you liked the garden furniture, made with gnarled wood, sculpted here and there with pixie and goblin faces.

BEN: Yeah, would look magical in our garden (far, far away Shrek look in eyes).

* * * * * * * * *

7.30 p.m.

BEN: What's up?

ME: I can't watch *Coronation Street* tonight.

BEN: Gettin' a bit much is it?

ME: Yes. Tina is in hospital in a critical condition, and Carla is blaming Peter for her fate. And Nick wants to divorce Leanne. So sad. *And* –

BEN: Never mind dear, *The Secret Life of Cats* is on later, with Martin Clunes. You like him. Cleo and Purrdi will enjoy watching it with you.

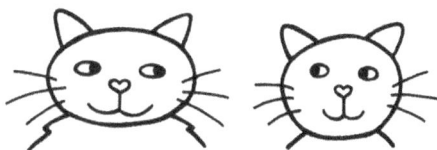

Tuesday 3rd

1.25 p.m.   My derrière was firmly seated on the garden bench, as I recalled last night's Chinese. I had tucked in, forgetting there were *root* vegetables in the tasty meal – I really didn't want to feel *grounded*. Yet. But my posterior was firmly planted. I felt heavy and rooted, like I would never *ever* move again (a common feeling when you have M.E.).

1.26 p.m.   Hundreds of tiny white roots were sprouting out of the soles of my feet, burrowing through my biscuit coloured slippers, into the coffee-cake-brown earth. Deep, deep, down among the wriggly, wiggly worms.

1.27 p.m.   Although I felt nicely planted, my mind was still away with the fairies. My head in the clouds.

1.28 p.m.   For some reason I seemed to see a lot of fairy cake shapes in the clouds (hmm, I wonder why?). A hippo with a dolphin's tail turned into a fox with a very bushy tail........ chasing a fairy cake....... A bat very .... slowly...... metamorphosed into an eagle..... a porcupine turned into a fairy cake............... a fish quickly became a crocodile with two humps on its back........like two little fairy cakes.

1.31 p.m. Fancy a fairy cake now. *Two* fairy cakes. Strawberry and lemon flavour, to give me a big sugar high. High as the birds in the sky.

1.32 p.m. Pity we've eaten the ones we bought at the festival. They were far too tasty, and light as a butterfly.

1.33 p.m. Now I see a fluffy, white dog with fairy wings in the sky, opening its mouth ever... so... slowly... about.... to... wolf... a... fairy cake.

1.34 p.m. I recall a couple at the festival who had attached pink fairy wings to their dog's back. It was a big black Labrador, and didn't seem to mind looking like a fairy dog (must have been a girl), although she may have been secretly thinking – What *do I* look like?!

1.35 p.m. Smiling to self. She *did* have a *very waggy* tail, and a happy dog face.

1.43 p.m. Ben sends me a text message:

IN SAINS – FANCY ANYTHING?

1.44 p.m. I don't hesitate to reply:

FAIRY CAKES PLZ X

1.45 p.m.   Will get back to my no dairy, no sugar, no this, no that, no the other, blah, blah, boring M.E. diet, when this stressful time with medical people is over......... one day.

1.46 p.m.   In the meantime, fairy cakes are the *best medicine*. Fairy cakes and laughter.

1.48 p.m.   I leisurely perused the pages of Joe Browns clothes catalogue. It was their half-price sale. The *Ocean Front* dress (with a swirly skirt) caught my eye – soft blue vertical stripes, with pink, orange and yellow wild flowers appearing to grow out of the hem. I could clearly visualise myself fluttering through frothy, white lace foam on a sandy beach, like a wild flower fairy. Enjoying the sea breeze ruffling my wings, re-lieving my wing-flop.

1.50 p.m.   Turned the page, and spotted a couple of shirts I thought would look great on Ben. The *Club Tropic-ana,* and *Beach Bar* short sleeved shirts, looked cool and colourful – with flower and palm tree designs.

2.00 p.m.   Leafing through a Woods Supplements catalogue, I noticed they had a sale too. I thought the summer weight loss section may interest Ben – for *after* his holiday. I dog-eared the pages to remind me.

2.03 p.m.   Tired of reading about the benefits of various oils, vitamins, and extracts of strange looking plants, I turned to a little more cloud spotting.

2.04 p.m.   A hedgehog with an eagle's head..... the head breaks off and becomes a fairy cake (surprise, surprise)...... the fairy cake stretches out...... looking more like an otter now, floating on its back down a river...... then drifts out of my sight. I start to feel like the sky – a little blue, with the promise of southerly winds.

2.20 p.m.

BEN: Here you are dear, fairy cake and a cuppa.

ME: Ooh. Now I feel in the pink, thanks!

* * * * * * * *

2.23 p.m. Ben joins me on the garden bench, fairy cake in one hand, coffee in the other. I can tell by crumbs on his lower lip, that he's already wolfed one.

ME: There's some supplements in the Woods catalogue that help you to lose weight. I don't suppose you're interested...

BEN: But you're gonna tell me anyway (yawning).

ME: Of course. Like the old bag Purrdi likes to play in, I can be fun *and* fascinating. Yesterday I was fun, hanging my fairy sculpture. Today, with the help of Woods catalogue health information, I will be fascinating. Well, a little. I'll be better on a good day.

BEN: Yes dear.

ME: Yacon root has been used for centuries in traditional Peruvian cooking as a natural sweetener. And it has recently emerged that it's a powerful aid to weight loss.

BEN: Marvellous.

ME:	Yes. Yacon extract is one of the best dietary sources of a type of sugar called..... hang on......... I'll have to read this from the catalogue... fructoo... ligo... saccharides, even though –
BEN:	Even though the sound of it is something quite atrocious..... supercalifragilisticexpialidocious!
ME:	Thanks Mary Poppins.
BEN:	You're welcome.
ME:	*Even though* these sugars can stimulate your taste buds, we cannot digest them, so they reach your gut intact. Once there, they feed the friendly bacteria in your intestine. This not only aids weight loss, but it boosts your immune system and improves your memory!
BEN:	Fascinating.
ME:	I like the supplement Garcinia Cambogia. Well, I like the *look* of the fruit it's made from – a miniature pale lemon pumpkin, with lime coloured flesh. Look.
BEN:	Very nice. Very witchy.
ME:	It helps suppress your appetite, and helps the body stop absorbing some types of fat.
BEN:	Magical.
ME:	And there's –
BEN:	Need the loo (hastily retreats indoors).

3.20 p.m.

ME: I've seen a couple of shirts in Joe Browns, I thought you'd like them for your birthday. Lovely tropical design. I'll get them a couple of sizes smaller than you are now, to give you incentive to lose weight. You've got till the twenty-sixth of October.

BEN: Yes dear.

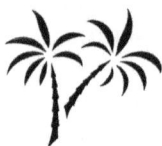

Wednesday 4th

11.30 a.m.   Wanda of Weekly Witch tells me Venus in Taurus, is in good aspect with Neptune in Pisces today. This means my creativity will be boosted. Hopefully my energy levels will be boosted too. I feel a *tiny* bit recovered from overdoing it a *lot*.

11.31 a.m.   Maybe I'll find the energy to *spend* time making a creative sandwich, with banana *coins* (for slow burning energy).

11.32 a.m.   Or do some doodling on my orange (energy giving coloured) post-it notepad. The sun is shining brightly after last night's rain, so I'll draw a smiley sunshine.

11.33 a.m.   Or arrange little yellow cups of sunshine in a wine glass.

11.34 a.m.   Or do an energy giving spell, to help me cope with my next appointment.

1.15 a.m.	I'm curled up on the sofa with my cats, full of banana sandwich (they are full of tuna), reading Celebrity Weekly. There are tell-tale crumbs on Ben's shirt (he is full of fairy cake).
BEN:	Nice flower arrangement (slurping coffee).
ME:	Thanks!..... Hollywood stars have been drinking green coffee to help them lose weight, *and* stay slim once the weight has been shed.
BEN:	*Green* coffee?
ME:	Yes. It's derived from the green un-roasted coffee bean. The extract contains chlorogenic acid, which is known to boost metabolism. It can trigger fat cell destruction in the liver, and inhibit the process of turning sugar into glucose.
BEN:	Great.
ME:	There's a berry taking Hollywood by storm too –
BEN:	Is that the time! Off to John's now, I'll be back in plenty of time to sort dinner.

* * * * * * * * *

4.20 p.m.	
ME:	Dear Great Spirit, thank you for bringing me in alignment with what I desire, which is for my highest good.
BEN:	What are you doing?

ME: I'm sitting on the lawn in the middle of a fairy ring of buttercups, with a lighted yellow candle and three sparkling citrine crystals. Oh, and chanting.

BEN: Who to?

ME: The sun.

BEN: Why the sun?

ME: It is the oldest, most powerful spirit on the planet. I'm doing a spell to to give me energy to go to my appointment with the osteopath. Hopefully he'll raise my energy levels. Then, after the appointment I'll make a complaint about the awful surgeon, *and* leave my doctor's surgery to join yours. I'm going to close my eyes now and hold in my mind a clear vision of what I want.

BEN: Will that include plain chocolate, or fairy cakes, or chocolate fairy cakes?

ME: I no longer hear you (eyes closed), I am at one with the Great Spirit. BUT before I am completely at one, YES to all three. *Well*, it *is* holiday time.

BEN: What *will* the neighbours think?

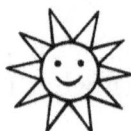

Thursday 5th

2.50 p.m. Ben returns from a trip into town.

ME: This looks a nice selection of musical veg.

BEN: Musical veg?

ME: Yes. Sugar snap peas, tenderstem broccoli, runner beans and peas. It says on the packet, Tender Green Melody.

BEN: Look again.

ME: Ah, Tender Green *Medley*........ Oh, and guess what?

BEN: Surprise me.

ME: I've just read in Weekly Wife, about a couple who are concerned about the health of their unicorn baby.

BEN: So people have unicorns for pets now do they? I *am* surprised.

ME: I should have read, they were concerned about their *unborn* baby..... I'd like a baby unicorn.

BEN: That doesn't surprise me at all dear. I expect you'd like a little dragon too.

ME: Of course.

* * * * * * * *

3.30 p.m. I forage in the kitchen for a chocolate fairy cake.

ME: Oh God.

BEN: What's up? Has your unicorn eaten all the musical veg for tonight's dinner? Has your dragon devoured the chocolate fairy cakes? Or burnt some toast? I did warn you not to use baby dragon fire for toasting bread.

ME: *He, he, he!* (big smile). You've cheered me up – now I've done my two smiles for the day. I'd forgotten about the two-smiles-a-day since we got back from the Faerie Festival. Mind you, I smiled enough on Saturday to last the rest of the month.

BEN: Yeah, but why the, *Oh God?*

ME: I was just having a moment of nerves about my appointment.

BEN: Next Wednesday?

ME: Mm (munch, munch) with the osteopath.

BEN: *Big Brother* is back on again tonight. That'll make you smile every day.

ME: Yes! Lots of people like me, sitting around trying not to go crazy. Tomorrow will be day one in the *Big Brother* house for the housemates. It'll be day fifty-eight in the Big Bathroom house for my mint plant, Minty. He's like a small bush now, and his leaves make a delicious mint tea.

* * * * * * * *

4.10 p.m.	I give Cleopatra a little groom, while I watch *Who Wants To Be A Millionaire?*
4.11 p.m.	I turn the volume down low, Chris Tarrant's quiz master voice is super-annoying.
ME:	Cleo and I have just made up a joke. What do you call a cat that's moulting lots of fur, and has inherited millions of pounds from its departed owner?
BEN:	Erm..... a very wealthy cat?
ME:	A moulting millionaire.
BEN:	Very good dear. You are fun today, will you be fascinating tomorrow?
ME:	Maybe. Wait and see..... Here's another one for you. I wondered why the frisbee was getting bigger, then it hit me.

* * * * * * * * *

9.15 p.m.	I'm engrossed in Channel 5. The *Big Brother* house is very different to previous years – minimalistic and futuristic, with bright colours. Not relaxing at all. This could cause some tensions.
9.21 p.m.	As I watch the housemates enter the house (one by one), I'm deciding who I think I'll get on with, and who I should avoid as much as possible for the next few weeks.
10.00 p.m.	I'm all decided. I will keep my distance from Tamara. She is a tough business woman who hates vegetarians and animal rights campaigners. I like Mark. He's

a slightly crazy scouser, dressed in canary yellow. His favourite subject at school was food. I think we'll have a laugh, and I imagine I'll get on with Pauline and Christopher too.

10.03 p.m. I switch the kettle on for a mug of *Snore and Peace* herbal tea.

10.04 p.m. I think I'll be best housemates with Helen. She loves animals, especially her beloved dog. Danielle is a strict Catholic. She seems nice, but I will avoid the subject of religion with her. Winston appears rather dim. But he once rescued a dog from a burning building, so now I'm in love with him.

10.07 p.m. Sleepily sipping my herbal tea, I smile at the next housemate. Matthew is handsome and intelligent, but I'm already in love with Winston. Although, if he (Matthew) gets cosy on the sofa with the pretty model (Kimberly), I'll probably get a little jealous.

10.10 p.m. Cleopatra snores on my lap. I don't want to disturb her, but I'm feeling the need to plod off to bed. I expect there will be someone with a loud snore in the *Big Brother* house, keeping other housemates awake. There usually is.

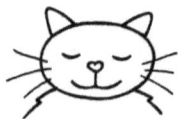

Friday 6th

1.00 p.m. I curled up under a blanket of warm cats, to watch *Most Haunted* by candlelight. Yvette and her team of ghost hunters were doing a vigil in a *most haunted*

300 year hotel in Cheshire. There were ghosts of a couple of monks, some poltergeist activity, and the spirit of an old lady. There was a spirit of a cat too, which was unusual. It belonged to the old lady and still follows her around. Purrdita and Cleopatra thought this was cool. So did I.

2.15 p.m.   Woke up after a little catnap with my girls. We all stretched and yawned together. They are much better than me at yawning and stretching – of course.

2.16 p.m.   I noticed the claws on my front paws needed clipping.

2.17 p.m.

ME: Purrdi, Cleo and I, just yawned and stretched at the same time, isn't that sweet? And the other day I scratched behind my right ear, at exactly the same moment as Cleo scratched behind her ear.

BEN: Was it her right ear?

ME: It was!

BEN: Marvellous.

ME: I've just had a dream that I was in the *Big Brother* house.

BEN: Did you have fun?

ME: Not at all. It wasn't bright and futuristic. It was a cold, dark and damp, haunted Gothic castle. All the housemates had been evicted to the dungeons, except Tamara the vegetarian hater, and me. She wanted to win *Big Brother*, so she decided to kill me, chop me up, and have me for dinner.

BEN: That sounds like a nightmare dear.

ME: Serves me right for nodding off after watching *Most Haunted*.

* * * * * * * *

2.30 p.m. Inspired by the haunted Gothic castle in my dream (and my creativity still boosted from Wednesday's celestial activity), I found my coloured felt-tip pens and Harry Potter colouring-in book.

2.33 p.m. I coloured away my cares, using energy giving turquoise.

BEN: That's an evil looking little goblin you've brought to life.

ME: It's a Cornish pixie from one of the Harry Potter films, remember?

BEN: Oh yeah.

ME: There were a few moments at the Faerie Festival, when I *really felt* like I was in a Harry Potter film. It was quite exciting.

BEN: When was that?

ME: About halfway through the evening, when I went off to find the toilets. I forgot it would be pitch black outside the tent. I could see a couple of portable loos in the distance, at the edge of one of the woods, because there was a tiny light. Then I started to feel a bit worried and scared.

BEN: You thought a wizard might jump out at you?

ME: No, I thought I might trip over a guy rope as I ventured between the tents. And I was a *little* frightened that someone might creep up on me, it was *so dark*. And I knew that after the tents, there was a small field, then a bit of a track to follow. But suddenly out of the darkness, some wizards and witches *did* appear from nowhere. They were a group of giggling children, dressed in long black cloaks and pointy black hats. One of them held an old-fashioned lantern, just like in the Harry Potter films, and the others followed behind. I hoped they were heading for my destination.

BEN: So you crept behind them.

ME: I did. And imagined I was with Harry Potter, and some of the students from the Hogwart's school of Witchcraft and Wizardry, heading for the edge of the Forbidden Forest. It wasn't hard to imagine because it was so cold, and felt creepy as we approached the edge of the woods. We had to climb quite a steep bank of gnarled tree roots to reach the loos, too.

BEN: So it was quite a little adventure.

ME: Exhausting, but fun!

BEN: So you'll be taking a small torch in your bag next year.

ME: No, you'll be carrying a lovely big old-fashioned lantern for us, and we'll take long black cloaks and pointy hats to wear.

BEN: Anything you say dear.

* * * * * * * *

9.05 p.m.   I'm glued to Channel 5 again, as five more housemates enter the *Big Brother* house. I think I'll get along with Ashleigh, Jale and Chris. But I'm not so sure about Marlon and Toyah.

10.05 p.m.

ME: I'm off to bed (big yawn).

BEN: To dream of little blue Cornish pixies flying around the *Big Brother* house.

ME: Probably.

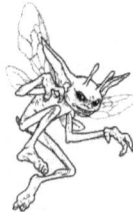

Saturday 7th

11.45 a.m.

BEN: There's a large parcel in the front room addressed to you.

ME: For me? *A parcel?* A LARGE ONE? (big smile).

BEN: Yeah.

ME: Goody! Can't remember ordering anything though (furrowed brow).

BEN: I think I know what it is.

ME: Did you have a sneaky peek?

BEN: No, I gave it a shake.

ME: So it could be in pieces now.

BEN: Yep, I think it might be (amused smile)......... I'm off to do the shopping now.

ME: Can you get strawberries. Wendy of Weekly Wife says they are in season now. They are packed with antioxidants, *and* a fantastic boost to the immune system.

BEN: OK.

ME: Wanda of Weekly Witch says the Romans associated the heart-shaped fruit with Venus, the goddess of love.

BEN: That's nice.

ME: Oh, asparagus is in season too. Do you remember I told you it's rich in folic acid? It's one of the vitamins your body needs to make serotonin, the happy hormone.

BEN: I'm sure you did. So that's strawberries and asparagus.

ME: And under-ripe bananas. They have a substance that helps you sleep.

BEN: Strawberries, bananas, asparagus.

ME: If you give me the list, I'll add them to it. I know your memory is getting as bad as mine.

BEN: Yes dear. Text me if you think of anything else.

11.55 a.m.   I text Ben:

             CHOC FAIRY CAKES PLZ

11.57 a.m.   I feel the need for a lie-down. Then fall asleep and dream of the woods surrounding the Faerie Festival. Although it's summer at the festival, there is a thick blanket of snow on the ground (dreams are like that). I watch in wonder as tiny dots of rainbow colours appear on the snow, like hundreds and thousands melting on a trifle. Bluebells begin to slowly emerge – their little blue heads sprouting through the sparkling white, the bells making a tinkling sound. Tiny Tinker Bell and snowdrop fairies, purple and green butterflies, and blue Cornish pixies fly around, giggling merrily. Bright, shiny red, perfectly heart-shaped strawberries, appear with golden-yellow buttercups. Asparagus tips shoot up. They are picked by the Cornish pixies, who are amazingly happy, because they are full of one the vitamins needed to make serotonin, the happy hormone.

12.10 p.m.   I awake with a little smile on my face, craving asparagus tips dipped in the cream on a trifle.

12.13 p.m.   Switch the kettle on.

12.14 p.m.   Tempted to send Ben a text message to pop a trifle in his shopping trolley. I'm sure eating a large bowl of sponge in jelly, with fruit, *and* custard *and* cream with lots of hundreds and thousands on top, would give me lots of energy.

12.15 p.m.   Can't find my mobile phone.

12.17 p.m.   Still can't find it.

12.18 p.m.   Oh well, that has saved me from devouring hundreds and thousands of calories.

* * * * * * * *

12.40 p.m.   Ben is unpacking the shopping. I watch for the entertainment. Cleopatra and Purrdita watch, to make sure the cupboard is being well stocked with tuna and Sheba.

ME: I don't believe it!

BEN: What?

ME: You got a trifle with hundreds and thousands on. *Just what I fancied.*

BEN: I've been telescopic! I got Fruits of the Forest yoghurts too.

ME: Mm... I expect forest fairies like forest fruit yoghurt and a pretty trifle. We must invite them to dinner!

BEN: Don't forget to invite a unicorn and baby dragon too.

ME: I imagine Harry Potter had *Fruits of the Forbidden Forest* yoghurt, at Hogwart's school of Witchcraft and Wizardry.

BEN: What are you like............. Oh, by the way, I'm going down to see Bill for a late lunch, as it's a nice day.

ME: OK. But Mercury is in retrograde with Cancer today. This can cause plans to go awry, so you must allow time for travel disruption.

BEN: Thank you dear, I will let Bill know I might be delayed.

* * * * * * * *

3.00 p.m. Ben sends me a text:

YOU WERE RIGHT - THERE WERE TRAFFIC DELAYS - BILL SENDS LUV - GOING TO ART EXHIBITION IN RYE - HAVIN MEAL IN THE MERMAID LATER - WOT WOZ IN THE PARCEL?

3.02 p.m. I reply:

YOU WILL HAV TO WAIT AND SEE - HAV A NICE MEAL IN THE MERMAID - LUV TO BILL X

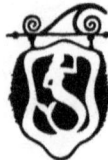

Sunday 8th

*There is nothing like
staying at home for
real comfort.*

JANE AUSTEN

A quote from *Emma*

8.20 a.m.   I'm eating a healthy breakfast. Three chocolate fairy cakes – healthy for a fairy who needs comfort food.

11.05 a.m.   I'm dozing under a blanket of warm cats – a comfort blanket for a fairy who needs comfort.

11.10 a.m.   I feel a poem coming on – therapy for a fairy who needs her mind taken off things worrying her.

COMFORT

*I feel comfy
In my slippers
I feel comfy
In my bed*

*And when I'm
Eating
Fairy cakes
I'm comfy
In my head*

11.20 a.m.   Still feeling poetic.

WITCHES EATING CHOCOLATE CAKE

There's nothing like
A comforting word
From your sister
In a coven
It can lift you
Like a chocolate cake
Straight out of the oven

11.50 a.m. Relaxing in a warm, Scents of the Forest, bubble bath. Fairies love a forest fragrance, and the comforting sound of tiny bubbles popping all around them.

11.51 a.m. I love the sound of the rain tapping on the bathroom window.

Tip
Tap

Tip
Tap

Tip
Tap

11.52 a.m. And the cold tap dripping, almost in time with the bathroom clock.

Tick
Drip

Tock
Drop

Tick

Drip

Tock
Drop

11.53 a.m.   Cleopatra sits by the bath. As water pours from the hot tap, I pour out my troubles to her.

11.55 a.m.   More verse pops into my head.

> *I FEEL*
>
> *I feel comfy*
> *On the sofa*
> *I feel comfy*
> *Under bubbles*
>
> *Makes you feel*
> *Much better*
> *When you tell*
> *Your cat your*
> *Troubles*

12.30 p.m.

ME: I'm gettin' really nervous about my appointment on Wednesday. I hope the osteopath is the same lovely, sensitive person he used to be. He may have had enough of his patient's problems, and secretly wants to kill them.

BEN: What are you like. He will be more experienced, so a much better osteopath.

ME: I'm sure you're right. A fairy loves comforting words.

2.15 p.m.   I'm watching a repeat of last night's *Big Brother*. The housemates are already getting very stressed-out. *Big Brother* has really put the cat among the pigeons, and a big, hairy dog too. I don't know why I watch this programme, it's rather cruel really. I'll blame boredom, and feeling lonely as a cloud sometimes.

2.34 p.m.   I'm SO glad I'm not in the *Big Brother* house, I can feel the **crazy** tension mounting. I am *most fortunate* at this moment, to be on my own with my purring cats – a comforting thought.

2.35 p.m.   And you don't feel so lonely when you are cloud spotting. You are not alone. You are one of the *cloud.*

3.00 p.m.   Gazing at a fairytale painting – Fairy of the Tides. It's on the lid of the large jigsaw puzzle box that arrived yesterday. I'm enjoying the enchanting fairy, colourful butterflies, reflections in the water, fairytale castle and foliage. I will make a start on piecing the border together tomorrow, when Ben is out. It will take my mind off Wednesday. Another comforting thought.

3.04 p.m.   Running my fingers through the puzzle pieces. A comforting sound, like the waves on a pebbly seashore.

3.05 p.m.   Spot two pieces of border joined together. I can see where they will go, they are part of a purple thistle.

3.06 p.m.   Ahah! This piece looks like a pale blue turret of the fairytale castle in the distance............ and this is the fairy's golden hair.

3.07 p.m. I think I will make a start. First I'll light red and white toadstool tealights, and place them next to my fairy figurines.

3.10 p.m. I sit, watching peaceful flames flicker on perfect little fairy faces, as they perch on toadstools.

3.12 p.m. I think I'll slice the last of the Portabella (fairy stool) mushrooms for a pizza tonight. *Another* comforting thought. Must remember to defrost pizza, so it cooks in *no time* and the mushrooms will not be over-cooked – their juice making the pizza taste (as Jane Austen would say) most agreeable.

> There is nothing like
> pizza at home
> for meal comfort.
>
> VERITY RED

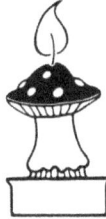

Monday 9th

ME: *Sniff..... sniff..... sniff.....* (blowing nose into kitchen roll).

BEN: Why are you crying dear?

ME: It's Peter Andre's fault. Him and his team of deco-rators, have just done a sixty minute makeover for a man with three young boys, who lost his wife to an illness. It's not just me crying, *everyone* is. Happy tears at the beautifully decorated home, and joy on the faces of the little boys. The man, his family and friends, are all wiping their eyes. As soon as Peter starts to fill up, that's me –

BEN: Weeping like willow.

ME: I can't help it, it's *so touching*.

BEN: Will you weep with surprise and joy if I do some DIY?

ME: I'll faint with shock (hand on forehead, eyes closed, head on one side).

BEN: That's not very touching.

ME: *He, he.* I had a touching moment at the Faerie Festival.

BEN: That's nice.

ME: Yes, it was in the music tent when you'd gone to get some drinks. The band had just finished a song and I was clapping. Well, you know it's hard for me to clap, so I was just gently patting my hands together, wanting to look like I was showing my appreciation.

BEN: Yeah.

ME: I was wearing velvety gloves, and the man sitting next to me noticed. He laughed, mockingly, and said I wasn't going to make much noise wearing *those* gloves. And do you know what I did?

BEN: Amaze me.

ME: I actually *replied*. Instead of sitting quietly feeling embarrassed, and wishing a sink hole would open up in front of me, and I could disappear into it. I *actually* replied, for the first time in the *millions* of years that I've had M.E.

BEN: I *am* amazed. It must have felt good.

ME: It did. I think the fairy mead gave me courage and energy. I wasn't a snail, retreating into my shell of self-protection.

BEN: You stuck your neck out and pointed your horns at him.

ME: YES!

BEN: What did you say?

ME: I can't remember *exactly*. I just told him why it was impossible for me to clap, even if I wasn't wearing gloves. Then I thought I sounded a little sharp, so I apologised.

BEN: You apologised! What are you like (rolling eyes).

ME: Do you know what he said?

BEN: I'm all ears dear.

ME: He smiled, laughed, and said he deserved it. Then we chatted like old friends – that's what I found touching. Then when you returned with our drinks, he offered you his wife's seat, because we'd only brought

one festival chair for me, and she was chatting somewhere else with friends.

BEN: Oh yes, I remember. Wizardly looking chap.

ME: He was. Very long dark hair and beard, with silvery
streaks. And little, wild, sparkly, bright blue eyes. I
think he may have been wearing a cloak. Can't remember.... There were funny, special moments too,
when I met some young fairies –

BEN: Is that the time? Must fly.

ME: Off to see Paul?

BEN: Yeah.

ME: How can you tell when a clock is hungry?

BEN: I've no idea.

ME: It goes back for *seconds*.

* * * * * * * *

3.05 p.m.   Posh afternoon tea. Earl Grey in a delicate Eternal
Beau cup and saucer. Two fairy cakes on a small,
matching side plate. Perfection.

3.07 p.m.   I'm leafing through TV Weekly, in a feminine-lady-
of-leisure way, wearing a fine cotton, cream top, with
tiny straps and delicate lace trim. My little furry-tail
princesses are purring softly beside me. I imagine
their diamond encrusted collars sparkling, as sun-
light streams through the sitting room window. I sigh.
Then smile at the title of a comedy film.

3.09 p.m.	We decide to watch *Garfield: A Tail of Two Kitties* at 3.15 p.m. on ITV – Garfield is mistaken for a cat who has inherited a castle.
3.22 p.m.	During the adverts, I find more pieces of the castle in my fairy jigsaw puzzle.

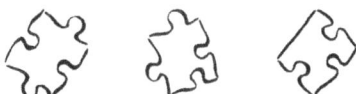

Tuesday 10th

ME:	*Eeeeeek!*
BEN:	You OK dear? I heard you screech. Big spider?
ME:	I'm fine. Just watching *Most Haunted*. Quite scary today.
BEN:	Ah.
ME:	The team is in Inveraray Castle library, doing a night vigil with their night vision cameras. A ghost is throwing books, and the cameras have caught drawers opening by themselves. Dead creepy.
BEN:	*The Ghost of Grenville Lodge* is on tonight. You can curl up with the girls by candlelight, while I'm out. Just off to Sainsbury's now, text me if you want to add anything to list.
1.45 p.m.	I text Ben:

FAIRY CAKES & FAIRY MUSHROOMS PLZ

1.50 p.m.   Ben replies:

FAIRY MUSHROOMS?

1.51 p.m.   I answer:

PORTABELLA - THE BIG ONES FAIRIES SIT ON

1.52 p.m.   Ben replies:

OF COURSE - SILLY ME X

* * * * * * * *

2.00 p.m.   Standing at the kitchen window. I nibble the last ch-
             ocolate fairy cake, and watch a squirrel nibbling on
             a peanut. She nibbles three times as fast as me, her
             whiskers quivering.

2.10 p.m.   Watching a repeat of last night's *Big Brother*. Things
             are getting so fractious, some of the housemates are
             about to explode again. They would feel happier if
             lots of fairy cakes were provided.

2.12 p.m.   I change the channel to watch comedy, and count my
             blessings I'm not in the *Big Brother* house.

2.13 p.m.   I count more comforting blessings and feel some
             verse coming on.

2.14 p.m.   *COMFORT IS*

             Chocolate
             Cosy feet
             Candlelight
             Coronation Street

38

Fairy cake
Fairy puzzle
Fairy pizza
Purring nuzzle

Warm milk
Teddy bear
Garden squirrels
Always there

Warm bath
Warm home
Warm man
Mobile phone

2.30 p.m. Sipping de-caf coffee and opening the pile of post I had forgotten about. It's good to hear from my witchy friend Jayne who has M.E. She is exhausted, and has relapsed after attending her sister's baby naming day, but apart from that, she's doing OK.

2.33 p.m. Received a beautiful floral card from my aunt too. She made me smile when she mentioned my uncle feeds a blackbird, who brings her two, fat fledglings to feed.

2.34 p.m. I count *more* blessings.

Nice people
Nice post
Tasty cuppa
Warm toast

3.00 p.m.

BEN: Why have you put the mushrooms on the window sill?

ME: They are soaking up magical sun rays.

BEN: Mushrooms like to sunbathe do they?

ME: Wanda of Weekly Witch says, they create vitamin D to protect themselves from the rays. So you up your vitamin intake when you eat them.

BEN: Genius!

Wednesday 11th

1.45 p.m.   Resting after my bath and hair wash. I'll be nice and clean and sparkly for the osteopath. To help me relax, I read one of my books about fairies that I bought many full moons ago.

2.00 p.m.   Purrdita and Cleopatra enjoy hearing a little poem, till their eyes go sleepy, and they drift off to feline dreamland.

THE RAINBOW FAIRIES

Two little clouds, one summer's day,
Went flying through the sky;
They went so fast they bumped their heads,
And both began to cry.

Old father sun looked out and said;
'Oh, never mind, my dears,
I'll send my little fairy folk
To dry your falling tears.'

One fairy came in violet,
And one wore indigo;
In blue, green, orange, red,
They made a pretty row.
They wiped the cloud-tears all away,
And then from out the sky,
Upon a line the sunbeams made,
They hung their gowns to dry.

ANON

2.45 p.m.   With a minty tea and fairy cake, I do some cloud watching. I see a hedgehog followed by two fairy cakes.

2.50 p.m.   I have another fairy cake.

3.15 p.m.   I attempt to tame my scarecrow hair with six hair-grips. It has been looking scarier lately, and I don't want to alarm the osteopath.

3.30 p.m.   We drive off to the clinic, my mood as light as a pink rose fairy, but a little anxious.

3.42 p.m.   I sit in the waiting room fluttering through the pages of an old, dog-eared Country Life magazine. Too nervous to read, I just glance at the photographs, not really seeing them.

3.50 p.m.   A door opens and the osteopath appears, wearing a white coat and a charming, friendly smile – good start. He doesn't seem to have changed over the past twenty-something years.

3.51 p.m.   John says I haven't changed *at all.* I suddenly feel twenty years younger – and I haven't had any treatment yet! I tell him he hasn't changed either. We laugh. Even better start.

* * * * * * * *

4.27 p.m.   The bright smiling sunshine, beams warmly at me as I leave the surgery. I feel light as a primrose fairy. A fairy who has been treated for wing-flop, and can feel her energy returning. Her damp, heavy wings are crisp and dry and ready to fly. It feels *wingfully wonderfully wondrous* to be alive.

I want to *BURST* into song (Julie Andrews style) about my wings being alive with the sound of music, and write poetry – all at once.

4.28 p.m.   As we head *laughingly* towards our car (parked just down the road), there's a refreshing gust of wind, followed by tapping noises all around us on the path. Then something falls on my head, startling me. Pennies from heaven? A little bird? No, it's a pine cone.

4.29 p.m.   There are many pine trees in neighbouring houses, and I notice small piles of cones littering the gutter. Although littering is the wrong word, they are not ugly, empty packets or plastic bottles. They are pretty, and inspire you to make an attractive centrepiece with red candles and gold glitter (and maybe a sprig of holly, laden with berries), for your dining table at Christmas.

4.30 p.m.	Sitting in the car, my wings neatly tucked under the seatbelt, I hold the cone that fell on my head, up to my nose. Then I breath in deeply.
BEN:	Are you enjoying a good sniff?
ME:	I am. There's a sticky substance where the cone broke from the tree, it *oozes* a fabulous pine freshness.
BEN:	That's nice dear (turning the key in the ignition).

* * * * * * * * *

4.35 p.m.

BEN:	You look *glowing* after your treatment.
ME:	I do feel energised!..... I poured my heart out to him about the insulting doctors and surgeon. He was very understanding. Especially when I said how sad I was that my old doctor had retired. He goes to the same practice as me, and was sad that a male colleague of hers had retired too. *And* he couldn't stand his new doctor either. We grieved together for a moment.
BEN:	What did he say about your hands?
ME:	He said it looks like I may have arthritis and tendinitis, and I should see a rheumatologist. He also said I was completely flat with barely any energy.
BEN:	I expect that made a nice change to being told how well you look.

ME: It did. I told him I felt flat as a sheet of wrapping paper.

BEN: Did he ask if you wanted to be rolled or folded?

ME: *Giggle, giggle......* He said, he thought it was best to give me just a little energy for now, and to come back in two weeks. Is that OK? Can you get more time off?

BEN: Yeah. So you're a lot happier now?

ME: Yes. But I was a bit embarrassed when he saw my scarecrow hair. While he was doing some cranial work, a few of my hairgrips fell out.

BEN: When he gave them back to you did he tell you to get a grip?

Thursday 12th

11.00 a.m. I'm smiling at the pine cone that fell on my head yesterday. I saw it as a sign of good luck. Like when a bird does a pooh on your head, but a lot less messy.

11.01 a.m. It is happily sitting on the kitchen window sill, with my fairytale collection of glass goblets, crystals, fairies, toadstool tealight holders, and a sleeping dragon.

11.02 a.m. I notice a tiny money spider has started to make a web between the cone and a fairy. Good excuse not to dust. And I like to imagine a feng shui expert would say; if a money spider makes a home in your kitchen window, this means there's a fairy energy flow, and one day you'll be able to afford a lovely new kitchen.

11.07 a.m. I smile again, as I notice a rubber-duck-shaped cloud floating across the summertime blue, when I wander into the garden to feed the wildlife. The collared doves are the first to descend, with beautiful out-stretched wings. I watch them flying above me, their feathers, the softest grey, and catch a tiny falling feather in the palm of my hand – light as a passing kind thought.

11.10 a.m. Back in the kitchen (feather resting on my sleeping dragon), I am at peace with the world, as I watch the grey squirrels joyfully scamper down from the trees for their morning feed.

11.29 a.m. Purrdita peacefully purrs.

11.30 a.m. Cleopatra playfully paws a piece of my jigsaw puzzle.

11.31 a.m. The clock...

11.32 a.m. Softly...

11.33 a.m. Tick...

11.34 a.m. Tick...

11.35 a.m. Ticks...

11.36 a.m. Morning...

11.37 a.m. Away.

11.38 a.m. I'm...

11.39 a.m.   Happily...

11.40 a.m.   Pick...

11.41 a.m.   Pick...

11.42 a.m.   Picking...

11.43 a.m.   Puzzle...

11.44 a.m.   Pieces...

11.45 a.m.   And...

11.46 a.m.   Watching...

11.47 a.m.   My...

11.48 a.m.   Fairytale...

11.49 a.m.   Puzzle...

11.50 a.m.   Very...

11.51 a.m.   Very...

11.52 a.m.   Gradually...

11.53 a.m.   Come...

11.54 a.m.   To...

11.55 a.m.   Life.

11.56 a.m.   Soft...

11.57 a.m.   Blue...

11.58 a.m.   And...

11.59 a.m.   Purple...

12.00 noon.   Fairytale...

12.01 p.m.   Castle...

12.02 p.m.   In...

12.03 p.m.   The...

12.04 p.m.   Distance.

12.05 p.m.   Vibrant...

12.06 p.m.   Golds...

12.07 p.m.   Reds...

12.08 p.m.   Oranges...

12.09 p.m.   Rusts...

12.10 p.m.   In...

12.11 p.m.   Fairy...

12.12 p.m.   Hair.

12.13 p.m.   Flowers...

12.14 p.m.   And...

12.15 p.m. Butterflies...

12.16 p.m. Everywhere.

12.17 p.m. Soft...

12.18 p.m. Greens...

12.19 p.m. Green-blues...

12.20 p.m. And...

12.21 p.m. Yellow-greens...

12.22 p.m. In...

12.23 p.m. The...

12.24 p.m. Rippling...

12.25 p.m. Water.

* * * * * * * *

1.30 p.m. I start to watch a repeat of last night's *Big Brother*. But very quickly change the channel. I'm feeling much too happy and relaxed to watch the housemates at each other's throats – they could do with some jigsaw puzzles to keep them entertained.

1.31 p.m. Cleopatra and I watch *A Place In The Sun: Home Or Away*. A couple are house-hunting in Devon and the Dordogne, France. We choose France.

2.50 p.m. A couple are house-hunting in Scotland and Spain. We choose Scotland.

3.14 p.m.   TV off. Just dosing. There's a man sitting in his car outside our house, speaking loudly into his mobile phone. He has his car door window open, and I can't resist listening to his conversation – it's so amusing. And I am a nosey person now.

3.15 p.m.   His accent is like a London East Ender.

'You alright mate?....... Not bad........ Yeah it was..... Don't 'ave much luck do I?..... Yeah..... Did you?..... Yeah........ Don't 'ave much luck do I?....... That was last week, it 'appened again today................ I don't believe it eeva!......... Even worse than last time!..... Don't 'ave much luck do I?.... Did he?.... Did she?.... Really?.... Don't 'ave much luck do they?.... Yeah.... Just like me mate!'

3.21 p.m.   He lit a cigarette, then had a problem starting his car. When the engine was eventually running; he had a lot of trouble trying to get out of his parking space because the cars in front and behind him, were parked *so* closely. I was tempted to open the front door and call out, '*HEY MATE! DON'T 'AVE MUCH LUCK DO YA?*'...... Ooh, I was *so tempted*.

4.00 p.m.   I'm being nosey again, reading the gossip in Celebrity Weekly. But feeling too tired to read much. So I mostly enjoy the photos of the celebs looking their best, at various award ceremonies and charity functions. And photos tweeted by celebs of their children. Peter Andre's is the best – him and his baby daughter Amelia, watching *Peppa Pig*. Danielle O'Hara kissing her little son Archie, and Alex Reid's daughter Dolly (dressed as a fairy) are both delightful too.

4.20 p.m.   I think I'd like a fairy costume for next year's Faerie Festival.

5.00 p.m.

BEN: Peter Pan pizza for dinner, followed by Tinker Bell fairy cakes, sprinkled with little stars?

ME: Magic!

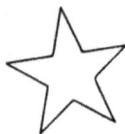

Friday 13th

ME: Last night's pizza was delicious. Why was it a Peter Pan Pizza?

BEN: Because it was deep *pan*. And I put extra green peppers on top, like the leaf green clothes he wears. Didn't you notice I cut the peppers in a leaf shape and arranged them in an arty way?

ME: Oh yes, *of course!* (hiding long nose). And I expect you flew the pizza around the kitchen a few times, before popping it into the oven.

BEN: Naturally.

ME: What are you like.

BEN: You. They say couples who live together for a long time become alike.

* * * * * * * *

ME: Do you like the pea pod boat in my Fairy of the Tides puzzle? Look, the fairies in the boat are wearing pea green dresses.

BEN: With pea green wings to match. Delightful dear. We're having fresh peas with the veggie-burgers tonight.

ME: Mmm.... I fancy fresh sprouts too.

BEN: You should read this book.

ME: Good is it?

BEN: It's *The Sprouts of Wrath* by Robert Rankin, very funny.

ME: I'll have a read when you've finished with it, it's a while since I've enjoyed a good bedtime read.

BEN: Where do books sleep?

ME: In a bookcase?

BEN: Under the covers.

* * * * * * * *

2.00 p.m. Ben plodded into town for some exercise, while I rested under warm, hairy, and purring covers, watching Peter Andre's *60 Minute Makeover*.

2.30 p.m. He sent me a text message:

IN SAINS-B – GOT BEERS – KITCHEN ROLL AND SPROUTS
– FANCY ANYTHIN ELSE ?

2.31 p.m.   I replied:

             `PETER ANDRE`

2.33 p.m.   Ben replied:

             `WOULDN-T YOU RATHER HAVE A HUNK OF CHOC CAKE?`

2.34 p.m.   I didn't hesitate to answer:

             `DOUBLE CHOC GATEAU PLZ X`

2.35 p.m.   Realised I'd forgotten to text that I wanted a *small* gateau.

2.36 p.m.   Shall I text him? No. I expect he's got the gateau already. He's probably chosen a small one. If he's bought a big one, then it means he fancies lots of cake for a holiday treat. So it won't be my fault if he consumes lots of unwanted-not-very-nutritious calories.

2.37 p.m.   I close my eyes and open my third eye. My witchy sixth sense is wide awake. What do I see?

2.38 p.m.   I see the colour purple. Has he bought plums?..... Purple cabbage?..... Aubergine?... Those new purple carrots?........ Purple serviettes? He knows I like the colour, and had admired the deep purple serviettes at an Italian restaurant we went to last year. Purple.... Purple...... Ah! Could be Cadbury's chocolate. He bought a very large bar for a colleague at work last week, who is going through a difficult time (he knows she loves Cadbury's chocolate), and I had gazed lovingly at it, after sniffing the wrapper.

2.39 p.m.   He will be at the checkout now, with beers, kitchen roll, sprouts, gateau, and possibly something purple. He will have less than nine items, so will be checking-out himself. Or be heading that way. He's a fast shopper. Hope he hasn't fallen and hurt himself, and *the something purple* is a bruise.

2.41 p.m.   It's most certainly far too late to text now, he'll be in his car. Or heading towards it. He's a very fast walker – may already be driving out of the car park.

2.42 p.m.   *Ah.* Just remembered he hasn't taken his car. But I expect he's plodding homewards with bulging carrier bags.

2.43 p.m.   *Although.* He may not have reached the cake section yet, because he has bumped into a mate he hasn't seen for *years and years.* And neither of them is in a hurry, and the supermarket isn't too crowded, so they stop and have a chat. He does *love* a good chinwag, especially with an old mate.

2.44 p.m.   *Or.* He may have been distracted by a three-for-the-price-of-two item, or a vegetable he hasn't seen before. He likes a bargain or trying a new vegetable. And the excitement of deciding whether to steam, boil, or roast the vegetable will make him forget the gateau.

2.45 p.m.   *Maybe.* The mate he has bumped into, suggests they have a coffee in the café opposite the checkouts. And while in the queue for a cappuccino, he spots the tasty looking cakes and remembers he forgot the gateau. *But then.* Decides he will get it on Saturday, because it will give me something to look forward to. And he knows how much I love something to look forward to, especially when it's food.

2.46 p.m.   And *I do love* something to look forward to, but all this thinking is making me crave a large slice of chocolatey heaven. Saturday may be tomorrow, but it suddenly seems *centuries* away. Fairy cakes are nice, but there's nothing like a creamy chocolate filling between layers of moist cake. I *truly think* I might die if I don't have a slice of *truly scrumptious* chocolate gateau soon.

2.47 p.m.   Shall I text him?

2.48 p.m.   Silly idea, he'll be in the door any minute.

2.57 p.m.

BEN: I thought you'd like the pictures on this kitchen roll, it's flowers in pots and a watering can.

ME: Sweet. I love the little pink and orange flowers, with the watering can watering the plants. It will brighten my day (one eye on the carrier bag that looks like it may have a box in it – one thought on chocolate cake brightening my day).

BEN: Do you like this purple cauliflower? I thought we'd try it. Looks witchy.

ME: Purple!

BEN: Thought that would surprise you.

ME: Yes, magical (hiding a witchy grin).

BEN: And I thought you'd like elderflower cordial. I remember you once said it tasted like a drink fairies would enjoy – it'll go down nicely with your fairy puzzle.

ME: Thanks! Sweet and magical (sensitive witchy nose trying to sniff out chocolate cake).

BEN: And.

ME: *And?*

BEN: They didn't have any small gateaus so I had to get a large one.

ME: *Oh, LOVELY!* I'd forgotten all about it!

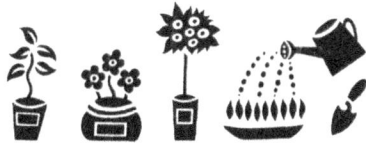

Saturday 14th

7.44 a.m.   I awoke feeling good after last night's pleasant evening – a double helping of *Coronation Street* with double chocolate gateau after dinner. And between episodes of the soap, fairy cordial enjoyed with fairy jigsaw puzzle.

7.46 a.m.   Then I remembered.

7.47 a.m.   Tonight.

7.48 a.m.   And sighed.

7.49 a.m.   And...

7.50 a.m.   Didn't...

7.52 a.m.   Want...

7.53 a.m.   To...

7.54 a.m.   Get...

7.55 a.m.   Out...

7.56 a.m.   Of...

7.57 a.m.   Bed.

7.58 a.m.   I...

7.59 a.m.   Just...

8.00 a.m.   Wanted...

8.01 a.m.   To...

8.02 a.m.   Lie...

8.03 a.m.   Dormant.

8.04 a.m.   Still...

8.05 a.m.   And...

8.06 a.m.   Flat...

8.07 a.m.   As...

8.08 a.m.   A...

8.09 a.m.   Door mat.

8.10 a.m.   With...

8.11 a.m.   A...

8.12 a.m.   Cat...

8.13 a.m.   Sitting...

8.14 a.m.   On...

8.15 a.m.   Me.

8.16 a.m.   Then...

8.17 a.m.   I...

8.18 a.m.   Yawned...

8.19 a.m.   And...

8.20 a.m.   Stretched...

8.21 a.m.   And...

8.22 a.m.   Fancied...

8.23 a.m.   A...

8.24 a.m.   Nice...

8.25 a.m.   Cuppa...

8.26 a.m.   And...

8.27 a.m. Needed...

8.28 a.m. The...

8.29 a.m. Bathroom.

* * * * * * * *

8.38 a.m. Switched the kettle on.

8.39 a.m. The squirrels usually make me smile.

8.40 a.m. But not today.

8.41 a.m. Why is it, when you start to feel better, you have to do something that stresses you physically or mentally, or both? *Why, why, why?*

8.42 a.m. If I don't go tonight, I'll lie around feeling guilty for ages. And that will make me feel stressed..... and..... I must have a nice warm bath to relax me – starting to feel tense.

10.35 a.m. Watching water drain out of bath. Will I feel drained after tonight?

10.36 a.m. Yes. And my wings might drop off.

10.37 a.m. BUT. I'm very happy I'm seeing an osteopath again soon.

10.45 a.m. Lying on bed and planning. Will lay clothes out ready (after lunch) and do as little as possible today. Will watch house-hunting programmes and vintage comedy – *Rising Damp*, or *Man About the House*, or *Bless this House*. Will eat energy giving bananas, instead of devouring the rest of the gateau in a moment of grimness. Will pace myself. Resting between dressing, doing make-up and hair. Will do a relaxing meditation in Weekly Witch.

* * * * * * * * *

11.00 a.m. I'm wearing my positive head. It will be lovely to be at a nice country pub – the one we popped into for a drink on the way home from the dentist last month. With the soft chairs and décor, and softly playing music. And when we arrive I won't be as *madly exhausted* as I was after seeing the *dentist*, and wanting to curl up on the floor and sleep with the big white friendly-looking dog.

11.05 a.m. I'll sip Prosecco while I peruse the menu. I will be calm and relaxed, and not strangle the person telling me how *wonderfully radiant* and *well* I look. And I will not throw a plate at their head, when they ask me what exciting things I'm doing at the moment. I will take a deep breaths, and hum along to the lovely songs playing in the background.

* * * * * * * * *

6.05 p.m. In car. Ben tells me to belt-up.

6.06 p.m. I do not want to belt-up, because I'm about to lie down on back seat of the car.

6.32 p.m. Arrive at dad's house.

6.37 p.m. Dad climbs into passenger seat.

6.38 p.m. Dad tells me *how well* I look.

6.39 p.m.	I politely tell dad to belt-up (resisting urge to strangle him with the seat belt).
7.00 p.m.	Arrive at country pub.
7.17 p.m.	I wish dad a happy Father's Day for tomorrow. We all smile and raise our glasses.
ME:	Did you like your card?
BEN:	I hope it made you smile.
DAD:	Ah, which one was that, remind me?
BEN:	The one with the photo of two characters from *Dad's Army*: Captain Mainwaring and Sergeant Wilson. The caption read, 'More chocolate? Do you really think that's wise sir?'
DAD:	Oh yes, very amusing.
ME:	Have a joke for you dad. A jump-lead walks into a bar. The barman says, 'I'll serve you but don't start anything'.
DAD:	Very funny dear. You *do look* very well.
7.20 p.m.	I smile, wishing I was at home watching *Midsomer Murders* with my cats.
7.23 p.m.	We peruse our menus.
7.25 p.m.	I search for the vegetarian meals, sipping my drink (that has gone down a little too fast). Oh dear. Now I will have more colour in my cheeks, and a sparkle

in my eye, and talk a lot, and dad might tell me I look radiant.

7.26 p.m.   I want to be at home, stuffing my face with chocolate gateau and watching *Death Becomes Her*.

* * * * * * * * *

8.30 p.m.   I visit the little girls room, while dad and Ben discuss sat-navs and serious stuff on the news.

8.38 p.m.

ME: How was your meal dad?

DAD: Very nice. Thank you.

ME: Your vegetables looked tasty. Cauliflower is one of the healthiest vegetables you can eat. Very nutritious, cleanses your digestive system, and heart chakra.

DAD: Heart what?

ME: Never mind dad – it's good for the old ticker.

DAD: The strawberries and ice cream were delicious.

ME: I read in Weekly Witch, the Romans associated the heart-shaped fruit with the Venus, the goddess of love.

DAD: That's nice.

ME: And in Weekly Wife, I read that strawberries not only have lots of vitamin C, they are anti-inflammatory, and good for your heart.

DAD: I must say, this pub does *hearty* meals.

BEN: I can see where you get your sense of humour from dear.

* * * * * * * *

DAD: You're looking trimmer, lost weight Ben?

BEN: Yeah, my clothes are getting loose (pulling at front of shirt). And I'm going to have to get some new trousers.

ME: He looks better for it doesn't he?

DAD: Yes dear.

ME: And you've got more energy. You said runnin' up 'n' down stairs at work is much easier. *And* remember decorating uses up lots of calories.

BEN: Yes dear.

DAD: All OK at work Ben?

BEN: Yeah. Just had a holiday. Back on Monday.

ME: You could do with loosing a bit of weight dad. Just loosing ten pounds will improve the health of your heart. It will also lower your blood pressure, reducing your chance of a heart attack or stroke. And you'll have more energy, because loosing weight reduces your heart's workload.

DAD: Thank you, that's very interesting. And what exciting things are you up to at the moment?

ME: I'm doing a fairytale jigsaw puzzle.

DAD: You weren't that keen on them when you were little.

ME: I have been learning to love them. Like herbal teas. Have you tried any herbal teas?

DAD: Can't say I have…… How many pieces?

ME: Pieces?

DAD: Puzzle pieces – keep up girl (Captain-Mainwaring-of-the-Home-Guard voice).

ME: Sorry, getting very tired. Five hundred.

DAD: That's a lovely challenge for you.

ME: Yes. Wonderful.

* * * * * * * * *

BEN: How was your beetroot salad?

ME: Tasty. Especially the big, fat chips. You looked like you enjoyed your spicy veggie-burger.

BEN: Yeah (sip…. sip). I expect you're more grounded now after all that root vegetable, and not away with the fairies so much.

DAD: She's been away with the fairies since she was a little girl, haven't you dear?

ME: Yes dad (sip… sip – feeling tipsy). Wanda of Weekly Witch says beetroot is sacred to Aphrodite, the Goddess of love, and it stimulates the heart.

DAD: Marvellous. Any other fruit or vegetables good for the old ticker?

ME: Apricots and pumpkin (yawning).

DAD: Do you still make a pumpkin lamp at Halloween?

ME: Ben makes it for me now.

DAD: That's nice. Do you go trick or treating?

ME: Did you say trick or treating?

DAD: That's what you do at Halloween isn't it? Pay attention girl (Captain Mainwaring voice).

ME: Sorry dad, getting sleepy. You're thinking of your granddaughter.

DAD: Oh yes.

ME: Ben found a recipe for pumpkin soup last year, it was delicious. We'll bring you round some, next Halloween.

DAD: Thank you dear.

Sunday 15th

ME: You feelin' alright?

BEN: Nope. Back to work tomorrow.

ME: That back-to-school-feelin' huh?

BEN: Yeah.

ME: Let's have some lovely comfort food tonight, with chips.

BEN: Good idea.

ME: We haven't got any frozen chips. If you take a walk to Sainsbury's, the fresh air and exercise will do you good.

BEN: It's pouring with rain.

ME: Oh yes. I expect it'll brighten up later.

BEN: I doubt it.

ME: You could join me doing a bit of umbrella spotting. Look, that man's got a big one. It's all the colours of the rainbow.

BEN: Lucky him.

ME: I've nearly finished my jigsaw puzzle, you could help me. It's a great feeling of achievement when it's completed.

BEN: The excitement will be too much for me.

* * * * * * * *

ME: You've got more holiday to look forward to this summer!

BEN: Yep.

ME: I see on the calendar it's Bill's birthday today. We sent him a card didn't we?

BEN: Dunno.

ME: I know we got one. It was a photo with a funny caption, like dad's card. But I don't remember writing in it, or giving it to you to post.

* * * * * * * * *

ME: Found the card. Are you poppin' down to see Bill today?

BEN: No.

ME: I'll remind you to call him.

BEN: OK.

ME: And when you do, can you tell him we got him a card, it'll just be late. It's the thought that counts.

BEN: Certainly dear.

ME: You poppin' down to see him next Sunday?

BEN: Yeah.

ME: I might come too, a bit of Hastings sea air will do me good. And Bill is very relaxing company.

BEN: OK.

ME: We could sit on the beach eating chips and pretend you're still on holiday.

BEN: If it's not cold and pouring with rain.

* * * * * * * *

ME: Here you are, nice hot coffee and a choc fairy cake.

BEN: Thanks.

ME: Did you call Bill?

BEN: Yeah, no answer.... I left a message.

ME: Did you tell him we got him a card?

BEN: Forgot.

ME: I've written the card an' put a first class stamp on, ready to post tomorrow.

BEN: It's stopped raining now. I'll post it on my way to Sainsbury's.

ME: Oh lovely, and the sun's come out!

BEN: Yipee (moody school boy face).

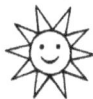

Monday 16th

6.25 a.m.   Lying awake in bed.

6.26 a.m.   Listening to birdsong.

6.27 a.m.   Thinking nothing much.

6.30 a.m.   Feel a poem coming on.

NOTHING MUCH

I'm doing nothing much
I'm thinking nothing much
I'm hoping nothing much
And wishing nothing much

I'm moving nothing much
I'm improving nothing much
I'll say nothing much
It'll come out double Dutch

So I'll explain nothing much
Or complain nothing much
Revealing nothing much
Or concealing nothing much

I'll peruse nothing much
And choose nothing much
I'll lose nothing much
And snooze nothing much

I'm planning nothing much
I'm scanning nothing much
Though I must write that letter
Nice to keep in touch

12.40 p.m. I send Ben a text message when he's at lunch:

I-M TOO TIRED TO COOK TO-NITE

12.41 p.m. Ben replies:

NO PROBS - FANCY A TAKEAWAY ANYWAY

12.42 p.m. We continue texting for a while:

ME: NOT BACK ON DIET THEN ?

BEN: NOPE

ME: TOO SOON ?

BEN: YEP

ME: I WISH YOU WERE STILL ON HOL

BEN: ME TOO

ME: CATS MISS YOU

BEN: GIVE THEM A STROKE FOR ME

ME: WILL DO - HOW WOZ YOR MORNIN ?

BEN: BUSY

ME: HOPE THE AFTERNOON WILL FLY BY

BEN: HOW-S YOR DAY BIN SO FAR ?

ME: GOT DOOR MAT I ORDERED - FUN DESIGN - UMBRELLA
          AND RAINDROPS

BEN: SOUNDS VERY YOU — I EXPECT THE CATS WILL THINK IT-S FOR THEM

ME: PURRDI IS ALREADY ON IT — WE ARE GONNA WOCH MIDSOMER MURDERS IN A MIN

BEN: I CUD MURDER A CHINEEZ

ME: TUNG TZENG HAD BETTER WOCH OUT THEN — HADN-T HE

BEN: HA HA HA

ME: WILL ORDER OUR FAVE DISHES

BEN: GREAT — THANX X

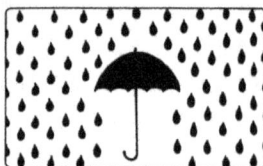

Tuesday 17th

7.10 p.m.

BEN: The umbrella and raindrops mat looks good.

ME: Yes. The cats like it too, they are taking turns to sit on it.

BEN: Doesn't surprise me.

ME: I finished the fairy puzzle, come and look.

BEN: Purrdi is sitting on it.

ME: That doesn't surprise *me!*

BEN: Cleo will be sitting on it next.

ME: I saw a fun cloud formation today. There was a boat-ish shape and anchor-ish shape. A plane flew by and left a white track, and it looked very much like a chain joining the anchor to the boat.

BEN: What a fun moment for you dear.

ME: Wish you'd been there to share it with me.

* * * * * * * *

ME: Got my newsletter today from the Kent and Sussex M.E. charity people. There was an article entitled, *Full Time Bird Watcher.*

BEN: That's you.

ME: I'd like to be a slim, full-time cake eater.

BEN: You could be a full-time cloud watcher or jigsaw puzzler.

ME: Full-time umbrella spotter on rainy days.

BEN: If we lived near a railway line you could be a train spotter.

ME: I'm a full-time cat stroker (stroking Cleopatra).

BEN: And daydreamer.

ME: I'd like to be a full-time practising witch, if I had the energy to do lots of spell work.

* * * * * * * *

ME: *Most Haunted* was really good today. The team were in Northumberland, at the Schooner Hotel. It's rumoured to be the most haunted hotel in Britain. It most certainly lived up to its reputation – *dead creepy* it was.

BEN: You'd make a good full-time ghost hunter.

ME: I would.

BEN: Although you haven't got much life in you to be frightened out of.

ME: True!

* * * * * * * *

ME: Peter Andre was funny today, on *60 Minute Makeover*. He was making a home lovely for a family in Hertfordshire. I really liked the room he helped decorate with warm reds, golds and browns. When he got covered in terracotta paint it was hilarious!

BEN: I'm sure it was.

ME: It's no wonder he keeps so trim, with his busy life and all that decorating.

BEN: Yes – little miss full-time Peter Andre fan.

ME: I used to be a big *Big Brother* fan, but I don't enjoy it anymore. The big boobed brainless blonde, who bobs around her bikini, annoys me too much. And all the fighting is too stressful to watch. And the latest task was horrible, using dead fish – as entertaining as watching paint dry.

BEN: Never mind dear, you are still a big *Coronation Street* fan.

ME: Don't feel like watching it at the moment. It was so sad, when Todd admitted to Tony that he was only interested in Marcus for his money. *Although,* it says in TV Weekly that Carla gets very drunk in tomorrow's first episode, and gets thrown out of The Rovers. So I may watch it just for that.

BEN: And you'll be hooked again. What are you like.

ME: An on-off *Coronation Street* fan.

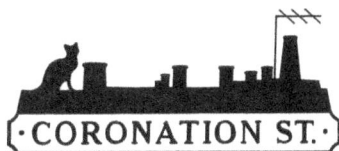

Wednesday 18th

12.46 p.m. I send Ben a text message:

I-VE BEEN A NORTY GIRL

12.49 p.m. He replied:

HA HA – WOT HAV YOU DUN ?

12.50 p.m.   We continued to text:

ME: I ATE ALL THE FAIRY CAKES AND HAV BEEN DRINKIN REAL COFFEE – SO I-M BUZZY AND HAV OVERDONE THE CHORES

BEN: SO YOU-VE HURT YOR PAWS AND YOR TOO FATIGUED TO DO DINNER TONITE

ME: YES

BEN: WOTS UP ?

ME: I-LL TELL YOU WHEN YOU GET HOME

BEN: I-LL GET A FRESH PIZZA AT SAINS

ME: AND SUM WINE PLZ

BEN: THAT BAD IS IT? – WILL DO X

ME: BIG THANX X

* * * * * * * * * *

6.20 p.m.

BEN: Here you are. Got prepared salad to go with it.

ME: Lovely, thanks.

BEN: Fairy cakes and wine.

ME: Even better.

BEN: And I thought you'd like these large picnic plates.

ME: Oh, they're delightful! *Love* the fairground picture and sweet, ice cream colours.

BEN: Nice and light for your weak paws.

ME: Paw-fect. Can you open the wine please.

BEN: Before it's chilled?

ME: Yes.

BEN: What's up then? You look like you've been crying.

ME: Oh, I got upset watching *DIY SOS: The Big Build*. Nick Knowles and his team converted a family's bungalow in Devon.

BEN: You usually enjoy a nice little weep dear.

ME: I know. But today's story was extra moving for me. The man was a music teacher, who was unable to care enough for his four little boys. He had to spend a lot of time working on the house, which was like a building site. And his wife had M.E..... I felt so sorry for the family.

BEN: Ah.

ME: It was very touching when *so many* people volunteered to help. And the family were *SO* overwhelmed with joy. Everyone was in tears. And the four little boys were *SO* excited with their new bedrooms.

BEN: And you felt *SO* overwhelmed with empathy, you ate all the fairy cakes.

ME: I only had one with a coffee. It was a letter in the post that made me feel stressed.

BEN: Here's your wine – bad news was it?

ME: Thanks – no, not *bad* news. Just, well....... I'll sort dinner and tell you later. I'm feeling a lot better already.

* * * * * * * *

BEN: What was the letter?

ME: Oh, I've got my appointment to see a rheumatologist.

BEN: That's good news isn't it?

ME: It is, but in the letter it says the whole thing could take two to three hours. It'll be exhausting and fatiguing. And the person I see may be as unpleasant as my new doctors.

BEN: You'll have to keep your broomsticks crossed.

ME: I will.

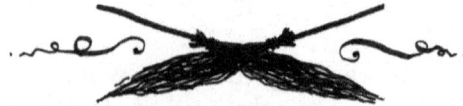

Thursday 19th

12.45 p.m. Ben sends me a text message:

HOW ARE YOU TODAY ?

12.47 p.m.   I reply:

BETTER THANX

12.50 p.m.   We continue to text for a while:

BEN: GOOD

ME: YOU MUST BE GLAD IT-S FRI TOMOROW

BEN: YEP - ARE YOU UP TO COOKIN TONITE ?

ME: NOT REALLY - QUICHE AND SALAD ON PICNIC PLATES ?

BEN: FINE - WILL POP TO SAINS - GET PREP SALAD AND HIGGIDY
          QUICHE

ME: SHAL WE BE GOOD AND NOT HAV CHIPS WITH IT?

BEN: YEAH - JUS PILES OF SALAD - I-LL GET BABY PLUM TOMS
          TOO

ME: LUVLI - SHOPIN FOR YOU - NO CHOPIN FOR ME X

* * * * * * * * *

1.05 p.m.   Switch kettle on, make an egg sandwich, and give my
            hairy girls a treat.

1.15 p.m.   Enjoying sandwich, and watching an episode of *Only
            Fools And Horses* entitled, *The Chance Of A Lunch-
            time*.

1.20 p.m.   Notice in TV Weekly, the episode tomorrow is the one
            I'm sure all *Only Fools And Horses* fans recall, en-
            titled *A Touch Of Glass*. The one where Del, Rodney

and their granddad, offer to clean crystal chande-
liers in a posh mansion. But the first one they start
work on comes crashing to the floor, and they leg-it.

1.21 p.m.   Recall watching a programme about the man who
wrote *Only Fools and Horses*. Apparently, the story
about the chandelier is a true one. I shouldn't smile
but I can't help it.

1.22 p.m.   Also recall the most enjoyable taxi ride *ever*. For
some reason the driver and I got onto the subject of
Only Fools And Horses. I think he reminded me of
the character Del-Boy. We spent the whole journey
laughing and saying to each other, 'Do you remember
the one where?' as he drove through busy traffic in
south east London, in a knowledgable way.

2.45 p.m.   Reclining on the sofa with Purrdita, after a most enjoyable time spent with Peter Andre. Today he was
in Northampton, doing his *60 Minute Makeover* for
a drama teacher who had lost her husband. He was
very hands-on with the wall papering (and woodwork)
and I loved all the dramatic colours, wallpaper designs, and striking theatrical paintings.

Peter amused the team of decorators so much with
his antics during the break, the designer (Ben Hillman) dropped his swatch, laughing. And he looked
so cute with paint on his nose – Peter not the designer.

At the end of the makeover, the drama teacher was
so *madly delighted* with all the bold dramatic colours
and designs, she wept theatrically, which started
everyone off. Even the designer wiped his eyes. And
as always, sensitive Peter was a little tearful. Bless

him. *And as always,* I had kitchen roll at the ready to dry Purrdita's fur.

* * * * * * * *

6.20 p.m.

ME: This spinach and feta cheese quiche is delicious, love the poppy and sesame seeds in the pastry. The salad is beautifully crispy, and so much more tasty when you don't have to prepare it yourself. *And* these baby plum toms are more flavoursome than the cherry toms. Don't you agree?............ It feels like we're on holiday, using these funfair picnic plates. We should have a picnic when you're next on holiday. I used to love going on a picnic when I was little, didn't you?

BEN: Yeah.

ME: I remember once, going to a Prince concert in the eighties, though I wasn't a fan. Didn't like his music much. Thought that *Purple Rain* song was boring, didn't you?

BEN: Yeah. Why did you go to his concert, if you weren't a fan? Is there a connection with picnics?

ME: I'll come to that. A boyfriend at the time, fancied Prince's female percussion player, and wanted me to go to the concert with him. And there was a new bloke at work who was going to the concert with his wife. He seemed a nice, friendly chap, and I thought it would give us something in common to talk about.

BEN: Did you have a picnic during the concert?

ME: We had one before the concert. Everyone sat in a field before going into the theatre. And I thought it would be funny to be among all the cool looking fans, and not be cool at all. It was the Love-Sexy tour, or something *really cringey* like that. So I dressed in a pretty, flowery Laura Ashley dress, instead of tight, sexy, pink and black Lycra. And I brought a picnic in a wicker basket. Then skipped joyfully to a nice spot on the grass.

BEN: I can see you doing that dear. You probably sang a little song as you skipped along, like Dorothy, when she's off to see the wonderful wizard of Oz. Except you were off to see a strange little man on a big stage, who was wizard on the guitar.

ME: Yes. Then I laid picnic food on colourful picnic plates, with picnic knives and forks, on a red and white check tablecloth. While the fans ate fast food and swigged out of cans and bottles, we tucked into our posh spread. It was more fun than the concert, seeing their faces. You can imagine can't you!

BEN: Like the time you turned up at a work colleague's posh wedding reception dressed as a witch, because she got married at Halloween. Fortunately the bride thought this was hilarious, and you had your photo taken together.

ME: I'd forgotten about that! The photo looked good. Her all in white –

BEN: You all in black.

ME: Anyway, I did enjoy Prince's percussion player, Sheila something, she was rather good. And a lot of work had gone into the presentation of the show.

BEN: Like your picnic.

ME: Yes! I had probably spent ages making coleslaw, preparing the salad veg, making a fresh fruit salad (to go with a variety of fruit yoghurts), veggie sausage rolls and quiche. Then popping it all in little Tupperware boxes, that I'd bought at a friend's Tupperware party.

BEN: Did the serviettes match the tablecloth?

ME: I expect so. We should get more of these picnic plates. So light to pick up. And they're a good size. Not too big. Not too small. Such a jolly funfair design. I wonder if you can get serviettes to match. Could you look next time you're in Sainsbury's?

BEN: Yes dear. You've been at the *real* coffee again haven't you!

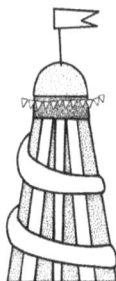

Friday 20th

11.20 p.m.   Where's my camera? *Where is it!?*

11.21 p.m.   When did I last use it? Got to get a pic of this to show Ben.

11.22 p.m.   *It'll be gone, it'll be gone. Quick! Quick! Quick!*

11.23 p.m.   It's gone....... It's a different shape now.

11.24 p.m.   Oh.... D**t

12.35 p.m.   Ben sent me a text message:

HOPE YOR AVOIDING THE COFFEE TODAY DEAR

12.36 p.m.   I replied:

I CUDN-T RESIST JUST HAVIN ONE - NEARLY GOT A GOOD PHOTO EARLIER - A CLOUD LOOKED EXACTLY LIKE A TEAPOT - THE SPOUT AND HANDLE WERE IN PERFECT PROPORTION - THERE WAS EVEN A LITTLE ROUND HANDLE ON THE LID - DIDN-T FIND CAMERA IN TIME

12.40 p.m.   Ben made me laugh with his reply:

GOD WAS HAVIN HIS MID-MORNIN TEA BREAK - WAS THERE A BISCUIT TOO ?

12.41 p.m.   I replied:

I WOZ TOO EXCITED ABOUT THE TEAPOT TO NOTICE IF HE HAD A SNACK - HA HA

12.43 p.m.   Ben made me laugh again:

ON SECOND THORTS - I EXPECT HE HAD ANGEL CAKES

* * * * * * * * *

12.52 p.m.   I'm sitting, admiring two paper napkins (it's amazing what makes you happy when you spend a lot of time alone). One is a beautiful deep purple, the other a gorgeous deep forest-green. I discovered them in a jacket pocket when I was hunting for my camera.

12.53 p.m.   Enjoying a pleasant trip down memory lane. The green serviette takes me back to a nice little pub by a river. There was a loch too. It was August. We sat outside having lunch, and I remember the bright pink flowers in hanging baskets, the lovely cool breeze, and groups of people gathered round small tables laughing a lot. Little birds fed at crumbs around the tables. Many of them were at my feet. They enjoyed quite *a lot* of my lunch.

1.00 p.m.   I'm off on another trip down memory lane. A lane with lots of interesting little gift shops, art galleries, and a church with a spectacular stained glass window, where I lit candles. A lane with many beautiful historic buildings, including a pub where smugglers used to meet. A lane with a pottery, a tea room where I enjoyed afternoon tea and scones, and an Italian restaurant (serving the most delicious pizza Margherita), where the cutlery came with a *purple* serviette, and a cute Italian waiter.

2.45 p.m.   Enjoying afternoon de-cat (I mean de-caf) Earl Grey tea and fairy cake, in my own little tea room (small sitting room), wondering whether to start another jigsaw puzzle, and wishing my short term memory was as good as my......... *sip*........ *sip*.......... *munch*.......... *munch*.......... what was I just thinking?

2.50 p.m.   I can't believe how absent-minded I am sometimes. Yesterday I found a tea towel in the freezer. And today

I poured half a bag of coffee into the cafetière, instead of the caddy.

* * * * * * * *

7.00 p.m.

ME: *I can't believe* how absent-minded I've become!

BEN: I know dear. I found an empty soup carton in the washing machine.

ME: There was an article about absent-mindedness in one of my M.E. mags. It was quite funny. A woman found a packet of smelly sausages in her shopping bag, and her purse was in the fridge. Another woman's husband asked her why her bra was in the bread bin. The mag asked people to write in with their stories of absent-mindedness.

BEN: You'll have to start making a list.

ME: I will! I recently found myself trying to turn the brightness of the sunshine down, with the TV remote control. And on the same day, I tried to turn down the sound of noisy children outside, at going-home-time, with the remote. *And* sometimes, I attempt to change TV channels with my mobile phone.

BEN: Do you try to text me with the remote?

ME: I have done (guilty-smiling-face).

BEN: I've seen you trying to change channels with the remote on your little TV, but can't because one of the cats is sitting in front of it.

ME: It's weird. I just forget for a moment, that the remote won't work through lovely, warm cat body. *Always* makes me laugh.

BEN: I'm sure Cleo and Purrdi find it amusing too dear.

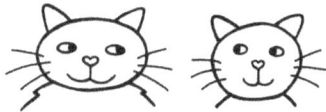

Saturday 21st

BEN: What are you doing on your knees, so early in the morning, lost something absent-mindedly?

ME: I'm saluting the sun.

BEN: Dare I ask why?

ME: Today is the witchy festival, Litha.

BEN: Litha?

ME: Summer Solstice.

BEN: Ah.

ME: It's a time when lunar and solar energies are at their height. Spell work is super-charged (bright witchy look in eye).

BEN: That's nice.

ME: I can't attend a Solstice gathering. So I'm watching the sun rise, and tuning in with the people marking the sunrise at stone circles. *And*, by the way, I am also on the floor looking for a baby plum tomato that rolled onto the floor last night, the cats must have been playing with it.

* * * * * * * * *

10.50 a.m.   Ben sends me a text:

IN SAINS - WONT TO ADD ANYTHIN TO LIST ?

10.51 p.m.   I reply:

APRICOTS - CARROTS - CIDER - ORANGE JELLY - MAN-DARINS - ORANGE PEPPERS PLZ

* * * * * * * * *

11.45 p.m.

BEN: Have you got a sudden desire for apricots, mandarins, orange jelly, orange peppers, carrots and cider?

ME: Wanda of Weekly Witch says apricots are in season. They are a good fruit to eat today because they are golden. I thought we could have mandarins too, because the colours of the festival Litha are orange and golden yellows. The God wears gold and the Goddess, red.

BEN: That's why you're wearing red today, and want to eat orange food (rolling eyes).

ME: And orange is an energy giving colour. I *need energy* to do a spell to *give me energy,* to enjoy an afternoon at the seaside tomorrow.

BEN: I haven't got a golden shirt (hand on head, very disappointed expression).

ME: But you can celebrate with me by drinking a golden liquid!

BEN: I got Strongbow cider.

ME: Lovely. Witches should have a picnic. I thought we could eat dinner off our picnic plates, sitting on the garden bench instead.

BEN: Anything you say dear.

ME: Can you make coleslaw with the last of the cabbage and lots of carrots. I'll put orange pepper in a sunshine design on a frozen pizza, and red pepper too, in honour of the Goddess. The pizza is already topped with golden cheese.

BEN: OK.

ME: I'll do apricot and mandarin segments in orange jelly. Hmm…….. maybe add strawberries. I'll need a hand with all the choppin' if you don't mind. We've got soya cream.

BEN: Yes dear. You've been drinking *real* coffee again haven't you!

ME: Well, I *was* up very early, and don't want to fall asleep in my dinner. I think I'll put a little golden eyeshadow on you, and you've got a lightweight yellow mac. We could sit on it, and I'll wear buttercups in my hair.

87

BEN: Will you invite the fairies to your celebration?

ME: Oh yes. The wildlife and our seven dwarves garden gnomes too.

BEN: What *will* the neighbours think.

* * * * * * * *

BEN: I got you two prezzies to celebrate Summer Solstice.

ME: Oh goody!

BEN: You can wear one in the bath.

ME: In the bath?

BEN: Yep, close your eyes and open your paws.

ME: I'll be opening my pores in the bath, *ha, ha.*

BEN: Eyes tight shut?

ME: Yes.

BEN: Both eyes?

ME: Yes.

BEN: Here's the first one.

ME: Oh, lovely honey (opening eyes with delighted smile).

BEN: You've never called me honey before!

ME: It's got *honey* in it.

BEN: Oh, I knew that *of course*. Something golden for your Solstice celebration.

ME: Honey and lavender *and* almond oil. My tired old witchy face will *love* a face mask. And the fuller's earth has a magical tightening action.

BEN: And as it's from Lush, so it's a fresh and organic.

ME: Smells *h.. e.. a.. v.. e.. n.. l.. y!* I've got a tube of apricot face scrub that was free in a mag. I'll use it before the face mask, and have the cleanest little witchy face for Summer Solstice.

BEN: Close your eyes again.

ME: OK (smiling).

BEN: Open paws.

ME: *Cackle, cackle!*

BEN: I thought you'd like them because they are cat eye sunglasses.

ME: Purrfect.

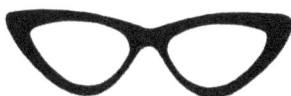

Sunday 22nd

BEN: It's a lovely day. Do you feel up to an afternoon sitting beside the seaside?

ME: (Bursting into song)

Oh I do like to be beside the seaside
Oh I do like to be beside the sea
Oh I do like to be beside the prom, prom, prom
When the band all play tiddley om pom, pom

BEN: That sounds like a yes.

ME: My energy spell work worked!

BEN: Great. I'll give Bill a ring, and he can wander down to the beach if he likes. You haven't seen him for years.

ME: That'll be really nice. I must remember to bring my cat eye sunglasses and a cushion, so I can lie down in the back seat of the car for the journey.

* * * * * * * *

12.56 p.m.   We sat on a Hastings seafront bench, watching children building sand castles on the beach and paddling in the shallows. I sighed happily, enjoying the breeze on my face and the sound of the waves.

ME: There's a fairy festival on in Cornwall this weekend. I wonder if some of the bands that were at our festival will be playing there.

BEN: Probably.

1.03 p.m.   Bill appeared, as if out of the blue, wearing black, and plodding in a weary Bill-ish way.

1.04 p.m.	After greeting each other, we all agreed it was time for some chips. And when Ben wandered off to the chip shop, Bill and I had a lovely long chat.
ME:	Alright Bill?
BILL:	Yeah.
ME:	Haven't seen you for bloomin' years, don't know how many.
BILL:	Ten.
ME:	Ten? The years have flown by *so fast*, like those seagulls (pointing overhead).
BILL:	Yeah.
ME:	Ben mentioned the seagulls used to wake you up early in the mornings, when you first moved down here.
BILL:	Yeah.
ME:	But you're used to them now, and they don't wake you up anymore.
BILL:	Yeah.
ME:	That's good. He said you had one nesting on the top of your wardrobe, in your attic bedroom. Is it still there?
BILL:	No.

ME: Ben said you were walking on the beach last time he visited you, and he was saying something uncomplimentary about the seagulls – and at that moment one flew over, and did a big pooh down the front of his jacket. It made you both laugh your socks off!

BILL: Yeah.

* * * * * * * *

1.07 p.m.   I watched a seagull nonchalantly plod towards us, and threw him some bread that I had brought to feed the birds. It was gone in a flash and we were soon joined by his mates. He had a lot of seagull mates.

ME: What have you been up to lately?

BILL: Not much.

ME: Did you enjoy your birthday meal with friends?

BILL: Yeah.

ME: What did you have?

BILL: Dunno.

ME: Can't remember?

BILL: Yeah.

ME: My memory isn't that good either. Ben told me you couldn't remember how old you were on your birthday. You thought you were fifty-nine, but your mum said you were fifty-eight, so you suddenly gained a year. Not as close to sixty as you thought you were!

BILL: No (half a smile).

ME: Have you done any painting recently?

BEN: Yeah.

ME: Ben mentioned self-portraits last time he saw you?

BEN: Yeah.

ME: How many?

BILL: Two.

ME: What medium do you use these days?

BILL: Oils... Charcoal.

ME: Lovely. Do you still go to life drawing classes?

BILL: Yeah.

ME: Oh good, I remember you used to enjoy them. Ben said you liked the larger, more well rounded models.

BILL: Still do (nodding).

ME: When I did life drawing classes, it didn't bother me, drawing naked women. But when I saw them fully clothed after the class, in the canteen, I felt embarrassed. Funny that.

BILL: Yeah (almost a *whole* smile).

ME: You've felt the same?

BILL: Yeah.

* * * * * * * *

1.10 p.m.   We stared out to the deep blue sea. Both deep in arty
            thoughts.

1.11 p.m.   Bill sneezed. I offered him two sheets of kitchen roll
            (with seaweed green fish design) that were neatly
            folded in my pocket.

ME: Nice fish design isn't it?

BILL: Thanks (blowing nose).Yeah.

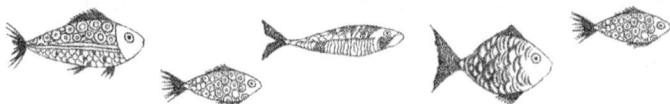

ME: I hear you did some decorating for your mum re-
            cently, which room?

BILL: Bathroom.

ME: Did you have a colour scheme?

BILL: Yeah.

ME: Sea view blue?... Golden sands?

BILL: No.

ME: Seagull grey?... Seaweed green?

BILL: Apple green.

ME: That's nice, I like apple green..... How's your mum?
            She always sounds so pleasant and cheery when
            she leaves us a phone message.

BILL: Alright.

ME: Ben mentioned she had gallstones, but has got them
            sorted now.

BILL: Oh, yeah.

                        * * * * * * * * *

1.11 p.m.   We watched a family wander by with buckets and
            spades, windbreak, and bags full of essential things
            for a lovely afternoon beside the seaside.

ME: Am I right – I think I recall Ben saying a while ago,
            you had one of your paintings exhibited in an art gal-
            lery here. Last summer wasn't it?

BILL: Yeah.

ME: A self-portrait?

BILL: Yeah.

ME: Well done, that's great!

BILL: Thanks.

ME: Do you ever paint the beach?

BILL: No.

ME: The fishing boats?

BILL: No.

ME: Hastings Old Town or the fishermen's huts?

BILL: No.

ME: The seagulls?

BILL: Nah.

* * * * * * * *

1.13 p.m. Bill lights up a roll-up and takes a drag, looking *artily thoughtful.*

ME: I wish I could have gone.

BILL: Where?

ME: To the art exhibition where you had your work exhibited. I would have said proudly to the stranger standing next to me, admiring your work, 'I know the artist!'

BILL: Oh (a *big smile*, looking chuffed).

ME: Ben said when he last saw you, you went to an art exhibition in Rye, by local artists. Was it good?

BILL: Yeah (nodding).

1.14 p.m. A family moved further up the beach, away from the incoming tide. I watched them slowly crunch their way through the pebbles, laden with deckchairs, picnic box, beach towels and an inflatable unicorn rubber ring.

ME: Are you moving house? Ben mentioned your mum was thinking about it?

BILL: Yeah (breathing out a puff of smoke).

ME: Seen any properties you like?

BILL: Nah.

ME: I used to fantasize about living on the Cornish Coast. But these days I'd be happy in a nice little bungalow on the Sussex coast. No more stairs. Heavenly. A bungalow would be good for your mum.

BEN: Mm.

ME: Will you keep living in Hastings?

BEN: Dunno (smoker's cough).

* * * * * * * * *

1.16 p.m.

ME: You've not been feeling up to much recently?

BILL: No.

ME: Seen a doctor?

BILL: Yeah.

ME: What did he say?

BILL: Not much.

ME: He didn't need to recommend lots of sea air.

BILL: No.

ME: But you need to cut down on the smoking?

BILL: Yeah.

ME: Carrying a piece of oak and a unicorn, I mean acorn, will be good for your health.

BILL: Why?

ME: In the Celtic lunar calendar, each month is influenced by the quality of a tree. Your birthday falls between the tenth of June and the seventh of July, so you are ruled by the mighty oak.

BILL: Oh, good (nodding).

ME: The tree was prized by the Celts, who believed carrying a piece of the wood or bark would boost energy levels, attract good luck, and help you achieve your goals.

BILL: Great (taking a drag of his fag).

ME: If I'm ever near an oak I'll get you an acorn or piece of bark.

BILL: Thanks.

ME: You look sunburnt on your arms.

BILL: Yeah (smokers cough).

ME: The Romans used chives to treat sore throats and sunburn.

BILL: Did they (coughs again).

ME: I like them in cottage cheese.

BILL: Romans?

ME: Chives (giggling).

BILL: Yeah, nice.

ME: Do you still love bananas?

BILL: Yeah.

ME: They're good for depression.

BILL: Good.

ME: Why did the banana go to the doctors?

BILL: Dunno.

ME: Because it wasn't peeling well.

1.21 p.m.   Bill nodded with a faint smile. I suddenly felt *very* tired, *very* hungry and a bit chilly. I watched a sandcastle crumble under rolling waves. Then I sneezed. Fishing another square of neatly folded kitchen roll out of a pocket in my handbag, I thought it had probably been there a long time (it was quite a while since I'd seen the beach hut design – very apt for a day beside the seaside). I showed it to Bill. We both smiled. Though I think Bill was showing delight at the sight of Ben approaching with three large bags of hot, fat chips – rather than enamour at a beach hut design on kitchen roll.

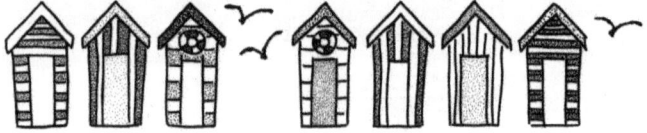

WE MUNCHED

ME: Noel Edmonds has a dog called Chips. Guess what his cat is called?

BILL: Fish?

ME: Yes!

BEN: Has he got rabbits called Salt and Vinegar?

ME: He may have! I didn't used to like him much, but he said he *really really* liked cats, in conversation with a contestant on a game show.

BEN: So you *really really* like him now.

WE LAUGHED

BEN: What did the ocean say to the shore?

BILL: Erm (*munch...... munch*).

ME: *Sea* you later?...... *Sea view* later?

BEN: No.

ME: Sorry I put a damper on things?

BEN: No (*munch...... munch*).

ME: Can I come in now?

BILL: (*Munch..... munch..... chuckle..... cough..... cough....
        almost chocking on a chip*).

BEN: I'm afraid not.

ME: You're a *frayed knot* are you? A piece of old rope
        that's *very frayed*? One of those nautical knots? A
        sailing knot, or maybe a fisherman's knot?

BEN: Very amusing dear. Keep guessing.

ME: Umm...... I'm gonna really splash out today?

BEN: No. Any ideas Bill?

BILL: Erm.... No mate.

ME: Sometimes I don't know if I'm coming or going?

BEN: No.

ME: I give up. What did the ocean say to the shore?

BEN: Nothing. It just gave a little wave.

ME: (*Munch.... munch...... chuckle.... cough.... cough....
        cough.... almost chocking on a chip*).

1.45 p.m.	Full of chips and feeling thirsty, Bill and Ben decided to go to the café they always go to, for a coffee. I needed a lie-down in the car.
BEN:	Shall I bring you a coffee?
ME:	I'm OK thanks, I've got a bottle of water in the car.
1.48 p.m.	I sit in the car, windows open, sipping water and watching a ship sail across the horizon.
1.49 p.m.	A little wave of inspiration gently splashes onto the pebbles of my mind.

Watching waves
Distant ships
Quenching thirst
As she sips

Wipes the water
From her lips
They were very
Tasty chips

1.59 p.m.	Sparkling white witchy waves of inspiration, curl and crash onto the soft sandy shores of my senses... then fan-out to form a fine... foam... filigree of ideas for *fabulous* spell work.
2.01 p.m.	I would love to return to a deserted beach sometime (at new or full moon), near Hastings, and perform a spell that heals old wounds and helps you make a fresh start.
2.02 p.m.	A spell that has its origins in the Norse culture, where diverse traditions grew up around the sea. I

will perform the spell at incoming tide – of all water magic, that which flows from the sea is the most potent.

2.03 p.m.   The spell won't be too tiring for a worn out witch. And all I'll need is two shells, a silver coin, some wine, and fresh or dried vervain leaves. I will ask Ben to see if he can buy me the leaves from our local garden centre, and white wine from Sainsbury's. I have a silver coin and some shells. If Ben can't find vervain, I'll go to the garden centre with him and see which herb *speaks* to me, as I visualise the sea – that's a witchy thing to do.

2.04 p.m.   When I perform the spell, I'll hold the silver coin, shells, and vervain (or a herb that speaks to me) in my outstretched hand, and ask for the moon's blessing. Then drink a toast to the sea and moon, followed by a rest, while my mind concentrates on my purpose. Next, I'll throw one shell into the waves, chanting my wish as I do so. Then with the other shell, write my wish and name in the sand, below the high tide mark.

2.05 p.m.   What do I do next?..... *think*..... *think*..... *think* – it'll come to me.

2.07 p.m.   Ah. I'll wrap the shell and silver coin in the vervain leaves, count seven waves coming in, then bury the bundle in the centre of my message. Then I'll rest and wait for the incoming tide to receive my wishes. As I wait, I will chant – *'Tide and time receive my wish, and grant me new beginnings'*.

Then we'll have chips.

2.09 p.m.   A huge wave of exhaustion suddenly engulfs me –
SPLASH! I need to lie down, flat as shallow rippling
waters upon a sandy shore.

2.10 p.m.   I close my eyes and begin to drift off, carried away by
a tide of tiredness, out to the deep blue sea of sleep.

2.11 p.m.   The...

Sound...

Of...

The...

Rolling...

Waves...

Upon...

The...

Shore...

And...

The...

Calling...

Of...

The...

Seagulls...

Ever...

So...

Slowly...

Fades...

Away.

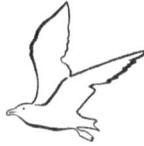

Monday 23rd

9.20 a.m.   Awoke with a nice little smile on my face, after pleasant beside-the-seaside dreams. I had *slept and slept
and slept*. An ocean deep sleep.

9.21 a.m.   Did I feel some verse coming on?

*Sleep, sleep
Ocean deep*

No. I was still in dreamlike state.

9.22 a.m.   Listened to my bedside clock. The seconds *tick, tick,
ticking* away. But I didn't feel my life ticking away.
Time didn't march ahead leaving me behind. It held
me gently by the hand, as we leisurely strolled along
a beach on the soft, warm sands of time, to greet the
day.

9.25 a.m.   Recalled some lovely verse my pen-friend Sarah sent me a few years ago. About a kind word, ripples in water and rolling waves. Well, I remembered the first line, as I watched the in-coming tide yesterday.

Drop a word of cheer and kindness

9.26 a.m.   Now I remembered two more. The last two.

Over miles and miles of water
just by dropping one kind word

9.27 a.m.   Decided to search for the verse, I really fancied another read. Sarah (who has M.E.) sent me the beautiful words to show her appreciation of my supportive letters. I was ocean-deeply touched.

9.45 a.m.   In bathroom, splashing water on my face...... Ahah! I know where it is.

9.46 a.m.   Brushing teeth, I feel some verse coming on.

Where's my verse?
Where's my verse?
I know!
It's in my mermaid's
Purse

10.16 a.m.   Sipping dark-seaweed-green minty tea and enjoying lovely words written by James W. Foley.

Drop a word of cheer and kindness:
just a flash and it's gone;
But there's half-a-hundred ripples
circling on and on and on,
Bearing hope and joy and comfort

on each splashing dashing wave
Till you wouldn't believe the volume
of the one kind word you gave.

Drop a word of cheer and kindness:
in a minute you forget;
But there's gladness still a swelling,
and there's joy circling yet,
And you've rolled a wave of comfort
whose sweet music can be heard
Over miles and miles of water
just by dropping one kind word.

* * * * * * * * *

11.20 a.m. Browsing through Joe Browns catalogue – They are having a half-price *SUMMER SALE*.

11.21 a.m. The little drawings of yachts, seagulls and clouds, are having a *SUMMER **SAIL*** across a sky blue hoodie. It catches my eye on the double page with a nautical theme. Lots of navy blue, bright red and white clothes and accessories. I love everything! Especially the *Ship To Shore Top* (blue and white stripes with nautical appliqué and embroidery), *On The Deck Dress* (sensational red and white stripes with sail boat motif), and *Bon Voyage Sandals* (navy with quirky maritime details and rope straps). But I especially LOVE the *The Lighthouse Hoodie*.

11.22 a.m. Have just noticed the little lighthouse drawings on the hoodie. It would be perfect for a breezy day by the sea. It looks summery and I could wear layers underneath. When everyone is in swimwear or tee-shirts, I won't have to look like an old lady in my cardi and jacket. I'll be warm, but look nautically cool, quirky and young – from a distance. I have some birthday money that I haven't spent yet. Shall I treat myself?

11.23 a.m.   YES!

11.24 a.m.   Beneath a photo of yachts sailing in a row, Joe Browns tells me to *plot a happier course through life.* I plan to do that Joe. I will start by ordering your light-hearted *Lighthouse Hoodie.* It will steer me in the right direction. I will be captain of my destiny. Standing with confidence, wearing my hoodie at the helm.

11.25 a.m.   A little nautical retail therapy does you good.

* * * * * * * *

12.40 p.m.   Ben sent me a text from work:

HOW R U TODAY AFTER YESTERDAY?

12.43 p.m.   I replied and we continued to text for a while:

SLEPT WELL AFTER ALL THE SEA AIR – BLEW THE COBWEBS AWAY

BEN: YOU NEED TO COMPLETELY REST NOW, TO SAVE ENERGY FOR YOR APPT TOMORROW

ME: I DO

BEN: WILL SORT DINS

ME: WOZ HOPIN YOU-D SAY THAT

BEN: IT-L BE LOTS OF ENERGY GIVING PASTA FOR YOU

ME: MAGIC

BEN: HAV GOT WHOLE DAY OFF TOMORROW

ME: LOVELY

BEN: I EXPECT YOR LOOKIN FORWARD TO YOR TREATMENT

ME: CAN-T WAIT X

* * * * * * * * *

1.20 p.m.   I curled up on the sofa, relaxing with Purrdita and Cleopatra, smiling as I read a lovely poem. It was written for me by my pen-friend Jim, who likes to collect shells on beaches in Scotland with his wife Pauline. He sent me a few tiny shells last year, that were *so exquisite*, I glued them onto a mirror frame I had made out of driftwood and shells, collected on Hastings, Broadstairs, and Whitstable beaches. They were the *perfect* little finishing touches to my creation, so I sent him a photo of my small masterpiece with my Christmas letter, and this inspired him to write a wee poem.

SHELL FEVER

I have been down to the sea again
The lonely sea and shore
I have found so many shells there
But I'm sure there's many more

The shells are very pretty
And some names are very cute
Like mermaid's bra and angel wings
Unicorn horn and pelican's foot

I sent some shells to Verity
And they're sure to bring her fame
Cos she used them with some driftwood
To make a mirror frame

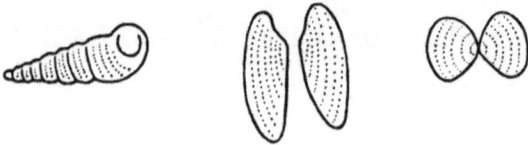

1.30 p.m.   There was a paperback sitting invitingly on the coffee table. I picked it up, and thought I'd have a little read before watching *60 Minute Makeover*. It was three books in one, by Jane Austen, that I hadn't heard of. Well, I don't recall them. I'm familiar with *Sense and Sensibility*, *Pride and Prejudice*, *Northanger Abbey*, *Persuasion*, *Emma*, and *Mansfield Park* – but this one was new to me.

Yesterday, while I slept in the car, Ben popped into say hello to Bill's mum. She was enjoying a peaceful Sunday afternoon, watching an adaptation of Jane Austen's *Persuasion*. Ben must have mentioned I was a fan of Jane's work, because she kindly gave him the paperback to pass on to me.

1.31 p.m.   I stuck my nose in the book. Literally. I opened the book near the middle and touched my nose between the pages. I love the musty smell of old books. And the biscuit coloured pages, that are so gentle on the tired eye.

1.32 p.m.   After a good sniff, I read a paragraph to see if I was in a Jane Austen-ish mood. I was. Especially as the character loved to be beside the seaside....

He wanted to secure the promise of a visit – to get as many of the family as his own house would contain, to follow him to Sanditon as soon as possible – and healthy as they all undeniably were – foresaw that every one of them would be benefited by the sea. He held it indeed as certain, that no person could really be well, no person (however upheld for the present by fortuitous aids of exercise and spirits in a semblance of health) could be really in a state of secure and permanent health without spending at least six weeks by the sea every year. The sea air and sea bathing together were nearly infallible, one or the other of them being a match for every disorder, of the stomach, the lungs or the blood; they were anti-spasmodic, anti-pulmonary, anti-septic, anti-bilious, and anti-rheumatic. Nobody could catch cold by the sea, nobody wanted appetite by the sea....

1.33 p.m.   I chuckled. I imagine they didn't have fish'n'chip shops at the seaside (to tempt your taste buds) in the late seventeen/early eighteen hundreds.

2.00 p.m.   Peter Andre was in my town today, on *60 Minute Makeover*. MY TOWN.

PETER ANDRE IN MY TOWN!

And not that far away (second big smile of the day). Only two streets. And one road. Near Mote Park. I can see the tops of the trees in the park from my bedroom window. Pete was near those trees! Lucky trees! Lucky family getting to meet Pete! Lucky house getting lots of attention from Pete!

Madonna did a concert in the park a few years ago, I could hear her singing. I shut the windows. Even though it was a hot day. If Pete did a concert there, I'd be dancing on our rooftop. Even if it was cold. And very windy. And raining, with thunder and lightning. Well, if I had some energy, and our roof was flat.

If the makeover show wasn't pre-recorded, and I was having a good day, *and* didn't have to save energy for an appointment or something, I'd be tempted to wander in *that* direction. I'd just happen to be passing by (with my camera) when the makeover was over, and a small crowd had gathered to clap and cheer.

At the end of the programme, the surprised mother of the family arrived in her car with a friend. She was confused when she saw the crowd outside her house, and a *very full* skip. But when she spotted Pete wearing his dungarees, *she knew*. Because she was a big fan of the programme.

CLICK! CLICK! CLICK!

I took mental photographs of the houses in the road (especially the makeover house). They were smart. Semi-detached. Neat front gardens. The makeover house had bright red garage doors. The woman's car was yellow. They had a black cat who liked to sit in the window. The house was number 9 – easy number to remember. I should have photographed the TV screen, but didn't think of it. Why do I often think of things when it's too late?

WHY? WHY? WHY?

I was tempted to wander over, just to be near where Pete had been. Maybe worship the ground he had been standing on, looking fit and tanned in his paint splattered dungarees. Maybe one of his empathetic tears had splashed onto the path. Oh, lucky path! A passing ant may have been showered by his tear. Oh, lucky ant!

I enjoyed an empathetic cry for the happy family, who were overjoyed with their brightly decorated home.

DRIP! DRIP! DRIP!

I especially liked the kitchen/diner. An interesting mix of whitewash and pine. Soft greens and blues. A feature wall with blue leaf design wallpaper. And lots of fresh looking leafy plants in pots. I just hope their cat doesn't try to sit in the plant pots to nibble the leaves, like one of my cats used to. There could be an interesting feature of muddy paw prints on the whitewashed dining table, and co-ordinating floor tiles. That wouldn't bother me, but it's not to everyone's taste.

I dried my teardrops on Cleopatra's fur with kitchen roll (a pretty fish design, in shades of green and blue). It would look good in the makeover house kitchen/diner. Maybe if I pop round with a roll for the family, they will be *most delighted* and invite me in to see their home. Maybe not. Not everyone gets as excited as me with a pretty design on kitchen roll.

6.46 p.m.

ME: You'll never guess who was in our town recently, near Mote park, doing a makeover programme.

BEN: I'm sure you're going to tell me.

ME: Peter Andre!

BEN: Great. I'm surprised you're not at the house now, peering through the windows.

ME: I made a mental note of what the house looked like.

BEN: That doesn't surprise me.

ME: Bright red garage doors. A yellow cat – I mean car. They've got a black cat with a pink collar, that likes to sit in the window. And the house is number nine. I thought maybe we could –

BEN: Drive past the house after your appointment tomorrow?

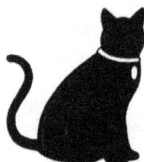

Tuesday 24th

10.30 a.m.

BEN: I'll do the weekly shop while you get your wing-flop sorted.

ME: Don't forget fairy cakes.

* * * * * * * *

11.40 a.m.

BEN: How did it go?

ME: Lovely. My wings are light and fluttery. I'll be doing lots of smiles every day.

BEN: Great!

ME: Can we fly across town now, for a quick look at where Peter Andre did his makeover? Just for fun.

BEN: So you can get out of the car and worship the ground he stood on?

ME: Maybe.

BEN: You should have brought your birdwatching binoculars, so if the family is out, you could have a peek in through the windows.

ME: What *would* the neighbours think!

* * * * * * * * *

11.55 a.m.

BEN: There's some red garage doors.

ME: *That's it! That's it!....* I think.

BEN: Yellow car in the driveway.

ME: Is it number nine? Haven't got my glasses on.

BEN: Yep it is. What do you want to do now?

ME: Don't know. Can't see much through the windows. Oh, there's their black cat with a pink collar, walking towards the house. I'd like to stroke her because Pete did, and I'll have stroked a cat touched by *Peter Andre!*

BEN: OK. I'll park.

ME: Only joking. It was nice to see the house though...... second thoughts, I would like to stroke the cat.

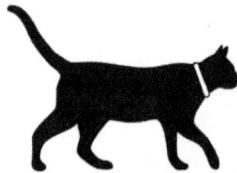

12.25 p.m.

BEN: Here you are dear, fairy cake and a cuppa. Good to see you with colour in your cheeks.

ME: I feel like a fortunate fluttery fairy. Do you know what today reminded me of, when you spotted the bright red garage doors?

BEN: Haven't a clue.

ME: Bright red rowing boat?

BEN: Nope, still no wiser.

ME: Norfolk?

BEN: No.

ME: Do you remember the calendar I got from the R.N.L.I. one year?

BEN: No.

ME: The one with the beautiful watercolour paintings of coastal scenes by Emma Ball. I think I liked them so much, I asked you to show them to Julia, who likes to paint with watercolours. Remember?

BEN: Oh yeah.

ME: And I thought it would be fun to visit some of the seaside places she'd painted, take the calendar, and see if we could spot the exact scene Emma had captured?

BEN: Yeah. That was years ago. We made the first one our summer holiday. We went to Seal Point on the Norfolk coast, and you loved the haunted coach house we stayed in. And before we went on a boat trip to see the seals, we found the scene painted on your calendar.

ME: We had hardly started to look, when you spotted the bright red rowing boat in the foreground of her painting. It was quite exciting!

BEN: Yes dear.

ME: Then, later that summer, we took the calendar to Broadstairs and Hastings. You spotted the big black lifeboat on Hastings beach in Emma's painting, when you were getting our chips.

BEN: And you spotted the beach huts in Broadstairs.

ME: We didn't go to any more places on the calendar after
             that. I know two of them were in Ireland. I remember
             the next one I wanted to go to had a lighthouse. I've
             still got the calendar somewhere, I'll have a look for it.
             Maybe this summer we could have another adven-
             ture.

BEN: Anything you say dear.

2.10 p.m.

ME: I found it!

BEN: Found what?

ME: The calendar with watercolour coastal scenes.

BEN: Oh.

ME: Look. Here on the back, there's two paintings with
             lighthouses. A black one at Dungeness, and a red and
             white one at Happisburgh.

BEN: I like the red and white lighthouse best.

ME: Me too, but Happisburgh is on the Norfolk coast. It
             would be a long journey, so we'd have to spend a night
             or two away. And we've already had a holiday on the
             Norfolk coast, visiting one of Emma Ball's painting
             locations. SO, I thought we could go to Dungeness.
             It's much nearer home. I looked on the AA map –
             probably take about an hour.

BEN: Dungeness is a desolate place. Miles of flat boring
             marshland in that area. And a gloomy nuclear power
             station.

ME: It's a wonderful haven for wild birds. It says RSPB on the marsh area of the map. I could take my binoculars and we could do some birdwatching. Maybe spot a Redshank, black-tailed Godwit, or a Great Crested Grebe.

BEN: Great.

ME: I could wear the lighthouse hoodie I've ordered. Look – here in Joe Browns (opening the catalogue at the nautically themed page), it's got dear little sketches of boats, seagulls, clouds and lighthouses all over it. Aren't they sweet?

BEN: Very.

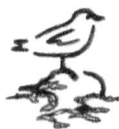

ME: There may be a page with a nautical theme in the menswear section, I haven't looked yet (flicking through catalogue).

BEN: Don't bother dear.

ME: This looks cool! (pointing to short sleeved *Tropical Pineapple Shirt*). Lots of big, bright, colourful juicy pineapples.

BEN: No thanks.

ME: *Hot Tunes Shirt* with melting records dotted all over it? Joe says when the music is on fire, you need a shirt that shows how you are feeling.

BEN: I don't think so.

ME: Funky *Flamingo Print Shirt?* The birds are beautifully illustrated, they look very real.

BEN: And very pink.

ME: Eclectic *Mexican Skull Print Shirt?*

BEN: No.

ME: Oriental tigers print?

BEN: No.

ME: Leaping leopards print?

BEN: No.

ME: *Some Bunny Loves You PJ Set?* Ah. I'm in the girlie section now.

* * * * * * * * *

ME: Looking closely at the Dungeness lighthouse painting, it looks like Emma was sitting or standing at her easel, on a patch of grass between two tracks. We should find that spot and have a lovely picnic.

BEN: If the weather isn't as dismal and cold as in the painting.

ME: How do you know it was cold?

BEN: It looks cold.

ME: Suppose it does really. And it looks like there's some smoke coming out of one of the chimneys. I wonder if those two chimney pots on the cottages *really are* bright red. I bet there're not. I've noticed from other locations we've visited, that Emma likes to use artistic licence to liven up her artwork. Can't wait to find out!

BEN: If you really must dear.

ME: Looking on the map, I see the lighthouse is near Rye bay. If the weather is very chilly, we could pop into Rye for tea and a scone, in one of the quaint tea rooms. OR, if I'm not too tired, we could venture in the other direction to Dover. Stop at Folkestone on the way for chips, then just view Dover lighthouse from the car.

BEN: Two lighthouses in one day! I'm not sure I could stand the excitement.

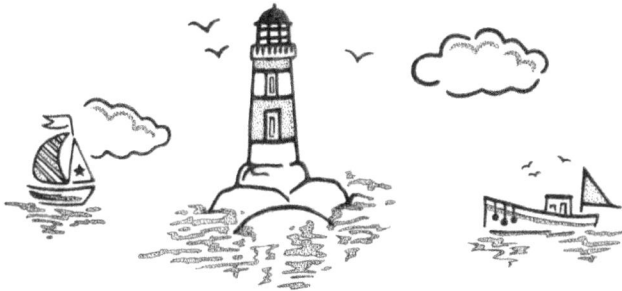

Wednesday 25th

7.24 a.m.   I emerged from under the bed covers and almost fell out of bed, feeling disorientated and a little dizzy after a stormy night. A night of thunder and lightning over our town, and in my dreams. Dreams that were more like nightmares really.

I was part of the crew on an old sailing ship, heading for Dover. It was an icy cold, stormy night. Sheet lightning flashed. Sails billowed. Joe (of Joe Browns catalogue) was at the hem (I mean helm), the ship's wheel spinning madly. His all girl crew were dressed in red, white and blue nautical fashions – Longline *Nautical Striped* sweaters, *Lighthouse* hoodies and *Ship To Shore* dresses.

As we approached the coast through choppy waters, I spotted Dover lighthouse flashing out of the blackness. Then the storm worsened. Rain and terrifyingly huge waves lashing the decks. The crew were slipping, sliding and screaming in their high heeled *Bon Voyage* sandals with rope straps, their summer sale fashions soaked to their skin. It was maritime mayhem as the ship rocked violently, and a mast broke with a deafening crack. I watched in horror as a massive sail fell, crashing to the deck, and onto my head.

I awoke to darkness, soaking wet and shivering, and slowly crawled out from under the sail. It was daylight. The light hurt my eyes. But all was not calm and bright. The crew wept below deck. Joe was still at the helm. And another storm brewed. The undulating waves, cup-of-tea-brown.

Were we approaching the white cliffs of Dover?....... No, a chalky white wall made of china........... Then I saw the bigger picture – it was just a storm in a teacup. A white china teacup in a saucer, on a linen tablecloth, next to a fruit scone on a dainty white china plate, in a quaint little tea room in Rye.

7.35 a.m.   My hot morning tea seemed extra comforting today.

7.36 a.m.   Fancied a fruit scone.

7.38 a.m.   Had banana on toast instead, and pretended it was a fruit scone.

* * * * * * * * *

2.01 p.m.   I sat in the garden feeling lovely and relaxed and peaceful. My dark green minty tea was a calm sea in a teacup.

2.02 p.m.   A small leaf dropped into it and bobbed like a rowing boat.

2.03 p.m.   Bees buzzzzzzed. Well, one bee really. One of the BIGGEST bees I've ever seen – must have been a queen. She looked very well fed and regal in her thick, stripy fur coat. And her buzz was *SO LOUD*, for one moment I thought a neighbour was drilling nearby. I was tempted to ask her if she collected nectar points from Sainsbury's. But that would have been silly – I expect her subjects collect them for her.

2.04 p.m.   Pink roses blushed. Birdies chirruped. My fairy sculpture, hanging from the bird table, slowly twirled and sparkled in the sunshine. A wee money spider dangled from my sun hat. A ladybird landed on my arm briefly to say hello, then flew away.

2.05 p.m.   I noticed I'd grown a few freckles on my arm. Minty the mint plant sunbathed his leaves. Blue and white butterflies fluttered at the end of the garden where the fairies live. I'm so glad we've kept some nettles to attract them (the butterflies *and* the fairies).

2.06 p.m.   I watched a single fluffy white cloud, wander lonely as a cloud. But it didn't look lonely when it met another cloud, and they sailed away together across the tranquil June blue.

2.07 p.m.   I sleepily turned the pages of Weekly Celebrity on my lap, just admiring the photographs and daydreaming. The ladybird returned, sitting on my hand to enjoy the pictures with me.

2.08 p.m.   We flew over snowy peaks in Switzerland, in a hot air balloon, enjoying a bird's-eye view of valleys, chocolate-box villages, and skiers whizzing down perfectly groomed slopes.

2.09 p.m.   Later, we would curl up on a cosy sofa by a warm fire at Le Grand Bellevue, near Gstaad. Apparently you can sometimes spot Madonna there on holiday. Maybe there are some sad people who go there, just in case they might see her skiing with her brood.

2.10 p.m.   I think, sitting outside a house, that has enjoyed a wonderful makeover by Peter Andre and his team, is not sad. *Noo.* Not if you live nearby. Two streets. One road. Nor is stroking a cat he has touched. Or, if you're a huge fan, worshipping the ground he has trodden on.

                I recall, the other day, on *Loose Women*, actress Linda Robson said she was a Donny Osmond fan in the seventies. She would follow him around the country, and one night after a concert, she picked up a KitKat wrapper he had trodden on. She has kept it in a safe place – there's devotion for you.

2.12 p.m. The ladybird and I are flying to Seville now, to stay at the Hacienda de San Rafael, with its all white exterior and beguiling ranch setting. You can sometimes spot Katie Holmes there. How nice.

2.20 p.m. Sipping a minty cuppa with a fairy cake, we're now flying off to the idyllic islands of the Maldives in the Indian ocean, to relax in luxury. I swim in clear tropical waters with the sea life, while ladybird sunbathes. If we're lucky we'll catch a glimpse of Victoria Beckham and her family. How wonderful.

* * * * * * * * *

6.30 p.m.

BEN: Today must have been boring after yesterday.

ME: Oh no. I spent the night on a ship in stormy seas. Then I had exciting adventures with a ladybird.

BEN: A ladybird?

ME: Yes. We flew over Switzerland in a hot air balloon, enjoying a bird's-eye view of the valleys, villages and skiers. And in the evening, cosied-up by a warm fire where Madonna stays on holiday. Then we flew to Seville, where Katie Holmes sometimes has a break. And after that we were in the Maldives, hoping to catch a glimpse of Victoria Beckham.

BEN: Very nice dear.

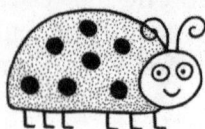

Thursday 26th

8.24 a.m.   I sip de-caf tea. Then smile. I'm re-calling last night's
            pleasant dreams. No stormy seas in a teacup. No crazy
            Joe Browns crew. Just me flying over tranquil seas on
            a bright sunny day. But not in a plane – on the back
            of a lovely ladybird, the size of a turtle.

            We flew at super speed across the channel, heading
            for Dungeness, then landed near the lighthouse, on
            the patch of grass between two tracks, where (I imag-
            ine) Emma Ball painted her watercolour of the light-
            house. In my dream the lighthouse was not black
            though, it was was bright red with big black spots,
            and we (the ladybird and I) agreed it looked much
            nicer than a plain old black lighthouse.

            On the patch of grass, there was a small gathering
            of famous people sitting on a rug, enjoying a picnic.
            Orchestral music filled the air from a small radio,
            the melody of Handel's *Water Music* gently floating
            on a cool sea breeze. Emma Ball sat with Peter Andre,
            Madonna, Victoria Beckham and Jane Austen. The
            ladybird and I landed nearby, and we were excited
            when they invited us to join them.

            Madonna was explaining the benefits of Botox to
            Jane Austen, who thought the whole idea sounded
            most disagreeable – Victoria Beckham's stiletto
            heels were *most unsuitable* for an afternoon by the

seaside too. Emma admired Peter's *60 Minute Make-over* dungarees and they compared paint splashes on their clothes. I felt inspired to recite a verse that popped into my head, about wearing dungarees at Dungeness instead of a pretty floral dress. Everyone clapped and cheered, and I felt famous for five *fabulous* seconds.

The ladybird lighthouse was a good conversation piece, and no-one thought it strange that I had arrived on the back of a giant ladybird. When Peter Andre told us a joke, we giggled like school girls, and Jane blushed as red as the picnic tomatoes. She had never heard such a naughty joke in polite society. Then she saw the funny side, and we all enjoyed a *most agreeable* afternoon by the sea.

* * * * * * * * *

12.35 p.m. I fancy a picnic lunch for one on the lawn.

12.40 p.m. Make a cheese and tomato sandwich.

12.44 p.m. Forage in the fridge for mini Quorn scotch eggs and small bottle of Scottish mountain water.

12.45 p.m. Open packet of cheese and onion crisps. Then place sandwich, handful of crisps, and two Quorn eggs on one of our large picnic plates. Garnish with peppery, aromatic watercress, spinach and rocket salad – sprinkled artily with leftover sweetcorn niblets, that look like buttercups nestling in the grass.

12.47 p.m. Sit for a moment, smiling at how lovely my picnic looks, and decide to have plump, juicy Scottish strawberries for afters. Luxury.

12.49 p.m.   Lay an old Stuart tartan rug on the lawn, then tune my old radio into Classic FM.

12.51 p.m.   Purrdita appears, plods onto the rug and curls up beside me, as I enjoy my picnic. She looks like she is enjoying the piano trio in G Major by Brahms.

12.57 p.m.   Purrdita is excited because she thinks Bach has written a piece of music with her name. But it is in fact, *Partita No 2 in D Minor.*

1.15 p.m.   I'm lying on the rug doing a little cloud spotting..... a ship with one sail...... followed by little fat fish..... and a treasure chest. Cleopatra appears and makes herself comfortable on my chest. She seems to like *The Blue Danube* by Strauss. Her whiskers and the end of her tail twitch to the waltz rhythm.

1.25 p.m.   Cleopatra enjoys the *Trout* piano quintet by Schubert, as she dozes off, afternoon sunshine warming her fur.

1.35 p.m.   I doze, listening to simple sonatas by Mozart, and feeling poetic.

* * * * * * * * *

3.00 p.m.   Peter Andre was joined by the interior designer Linda Barker today. Lucky Linda. She flirted with Pete. I used to like her.

             Pete, Linda, and their team of decorators, gave a lounge, diner and kitchen, a garden themed make-over, to a (nature loving) mother and her two daughters – lots of natural shades of browns and greens, reminding me of the jacket I wore to the forest themed Faerie Festival.

There were fern design blinds, walls and curtains, a petal lampshade, and rattan furniture. Pete potted ferns in terracotta pots, firmly patting the earth down with his strong hands. Linda flitted about in a panic, squawking orders like – 'WE NEED SOME HELP HERE!' – 'NO CUSHIONS AT ANGLES!' – 'GET RID OF THAT!' – 'YOU'VE GOT FIVE SECONDS BEFORE I BLOW THE WHISTLE!' – 'NO NOT THERE, *THERE!*' – 'NOT THAT HIGH, *LOWER! LOWER!*' – 'COME ON GUYS, **LIFT!**' – 'WHERE ARE THE INSTRUCTIONS?' – 'NO INSTRUC-TIONS!' – 'WE NEED MORE SHELVES!' 'WHERE ARE THE SHELVES?!'

As Linda's surname is Barker, maybe I should have said she barked orders. But no. She was a squawker.

It was fun to sit peacefully, watching all the noise and mayhem finally come together (pots and pictures perfectly placed), revealing wonderfully transformed rooms, ready to be admired. I particularly liked the fern design feature wall, and table made from tree branches glued together. But I think they should have included some fairy ornaments, and toadstool tea-lights flickering in the lounge corner, for a little wood-land magic. And the table was not as fabulous as the furniture made from gnarled trees, carved with little pixie and goblin faces, at the Faerie Festival.

4.00 p.m. After an enjoyable weep at the end of the programme, it was time for a fairy cake and de-caf coffee with Cleopatra, to recover from all the excitement and emotion. I dozed off for a while and had a pleasant little dream – Peter Andre and his decorators popped round to decorate my home, inspired by my fairy-tale ornaments and candles. Lovely.

5.00 p.m.   My kitchen did not look lovely. I covered the cooker with a clean tea towel (a green, leaf design, that Linda Barker would approve of). It was an instant transformation without the effort of cleaning.

5.01 p.m.   I lit red and white fairy mushroom tealights in the window, with my fairytale figurines, to create a warm glow, bringing the fairy faces to life. And making the dust less noticeable.

5.05 p.m.   I gulped a *real* coffee to perk me up, so I could do some washing-up. Then a little cleaning and tidying of worktops, and (armed with pieces of damp kitchen roll) I crawled on the floor, wiping the areas near the worktops.

5.20 p.m.   I absent-mindedly put a box of matches in the fridge, and left it there to amuse Ben.

5.30 p.m.   I found myself about to dry my hands on a slice of toast. Like the time I dried my fingers on a fresh teabag. Oh well, they *are* both *rectangle-ish* things that soak up moisture. Although I'm not sure why I would put a box of matches in the fridge.

5.35 p.m.   I added two more things to my list of absent-minded things I'd done, to send to an M.E. mag – it would give their readers a laugh.

* * * * * * * *

6.30 p.m.

BEN: Kitchen looks nice. Had another good day?

ME: Yes, I tried not to overdo it. And I wrote some verse, inspired by my dreams.

A LADYBIRD

A ladybird and me
Flew over deep blue seas
To join celebrities
For bread and wine
And cheese

BEN: Very nice dear.

ME: Peter Andre's makeover inspired me too.

60 MINUTE MAKEOVER

Higher, higher, lower, lift!
Now there's the sofa, just to shift!
Ferns and fittings well displayed
Carpets are no longer frayed

Oh, *and* my picnic, listening to Classic FM, inspired me lots.

LUNCH WITH MOZART

I love a good sonata
And a nice home grown tomata

Fresh cottage cheese is heaven
Like sonata number seven
Mozart adds a touch of class
As I sit upon the grass

Bird wings flutter in the trees

Like his touch on piano keys

BEN: Great. Do I inspire you?

ME: Of course (*think, think, quick, quick* – I must head to the kitchen for real coffee and square of plain choc to oil my creative cogs).

BEN COMES HOME

Ben comes home
For his dinner
On his diet
Gettin' thinner

Loves his TV
And his cats
Now avoids
Most types of fats

Also avoids
D I Y
Can be rather
Housework shy

BEN: *Ha, ha, ha* – that's me!

ME: I'm on a roll now.

Likes to strum
On his guitar
And pick at pickles
From a jar

He's happy when
It's time for bed

So he can rest
His weary head

BEN: *MY* verse is the longest, *SO* I inspire you more than Peter Andre and Mozart!

ME: Of course dear (secretive witchy smile).

* * * * * * * *

BEN: What's that you're humming? Sounds familiar.

ME: *The Blue Danube* by Strauss. Cleo liked it.

BEN: I thought she'd prefer Purr-cell.

ME: *Cleo likes a bit of Strauss*
Though she'd rather catch a mouse

BEN: I expect she'd like *Die Fleder-mouse!*

ME: Do you remember that dear little old ginger cat we took in? I called him Claude. You called him Claude de-pussy.

BEN: Yeah (head in fridge). Why is there a box of matches in the fridge dear?

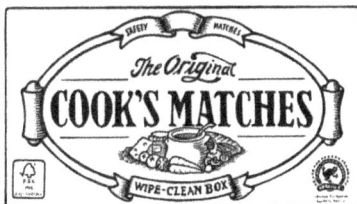

Friday 27th

12.10 p.m.   Purrdita, Cleopatra and I, enjoyed lunch al fresco again with Classic FM. We listened to music by Franz Liszt, Frédéric Chopin, and Henry Purcell.

PURRDI: Purr-cell is my favourite composer (cat language).

CLEO: Oh, I much prefer Strauss (cat language).

* * * * * * * * *

1.25 p.m.   After giving the bathroom a bit of attention (cleaned toothpaste spots off mirror, put out fresh towels and loo roll, watered the plants, and wiped a shelf), I put my feet up for a *well earned* rest. My feet were happy feet in comfy slippers. They felt smug, as I read about celebrity problem feet (in Celebrity Weekly), because my feet are *very comfy* every day, even on the rare occasion I leave the house in flat footwear.

The article was about foot care *really*, but a few celebs were mentioned. Victoria Beckham has bunions. That doesn't surprise me at all. Her feet often look painfully squashed into high, pointy fashionable shoes. They are not kind to toes, but are fine to wear if you are riding on a broomstick, because your feet dangle. Although it is easy to lose a shoe if you are not careful. And it is *so embarrassing* to have to knock on someone's door to say, 'Excuse me, I'm sorry to bother you. No, I'm not selling anything. No, I'm not a Jehovah's Witness or a moron, I mean a Mormon. I just think one of my stilettos has fallen down your chimney pot, and the other one has landed in your fish pond'.

Gwyneth Paltrow has bunions as well, and Elizabeth Hurley has cracked heels – they looked horrible in the photo. And there was quite a shocking photo of Kate Moss's toes looking red and badly deformed, squeezed into designer shoes. My feet felt sore just looking at it. But Sarah Jessica-Parker's comment made me quietly cackle to myself.

She was quoted saying, 'For ten years I literally ran in heels. I worked eighteen hour days and never took them off. My feet took me all over the world, but eventually they were like – 'YOU KNOW WHAT, WE ARE REALLY TIRED. CAN YOU JUST STOP. AND DON'T PUT CHEAP SHOES ON US!'

1.45 p.m.   In Weekly Wife, Wendy said that the British weather might not result in lush and exotic flora, but that doesn't mean we can't inject some rainforest razz-matazz into our wardrobe. I liked the tropical palm-print dress from Warehouse, and the mono palm-print top from Oasis. And I thought the Hawaiian Gandy's flip-flops would be perfect, for all those celebs with worn out, sad feet.

2.00 p.m.   Peter Andre was in Cambridgeshire today. He teamed up with designer Ben Hillman, to transform the Huntingdon home of an entrepreneur into a tropical paradise. There were lots of bold bright prints on walls and curtains, with a Caribbean look – lime green, cerise, summer-sky-blue, and sea-greens. Parrot prints. Carved drift wood. Paintings of palm trees with a hot-orange-pink background. Banana-yellow, purple and bright red candle holders. Metallic fish and carved coconut artwork.

Peter loved the pineapple print cushions. I loved the paintings of palm trees, coconut artwork, and banana-yellow candle holders. But all the *tropicallity* made me thirsty for a chilled, very fruity drink. And what I call a *narni-sarni*.

5.20 p.m.   Ben sends me a text message:

POPIN TO SAINS ON WAY HOME - FANCY ANYTHIN ?

5.22 p.m.   I reply:

BANANAS - PETER ANDRE - TROPICAL FRUIT DRINK

6.05 p.m.   Ben sends a text from Sainsbury's:

GOT BANANAS - I TAKE IT U DIDN-T WANT FIZZY POP - THE POP SINGERS WERE OUT OF STOCK - HAHA - DOES A BLEND OF PINEAPPLE, MANGO, ORANGE, APPLE, BANANA AND PASSION FRUIT SOUND OK?

6.07 p.m.   I replied:

SOUNDS LIKE A TASTE OF PARADISE X

6.09 p.m.   Then as an afterthought I texted:

CAN YOU ADD SUMTHIN ELSE TO YOR CHOPIN LISZT

6.11 p.m.   I could *see* Ben smiling as he replied:

WOULD THAT BE A BOX OF MINTY CONCERTOS ?

6.13 p.m.   I replied:

YES PLZ - AND A CAN OF SONATA SOUP X

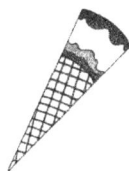

Saturday 28th

9.34 a.m.

ME: It's Mazey Day today!

BEN: Daisy Day?

ME: MAZEY.

BEN: Mazey Day? Amaze me.

ME: There's a photo in Weekly Witch. Look, what does it remind you of?

BEN: People dressed as green pixies – a fairy festival?

ME: It reminds me of that too. But it's a *much* bigger event in Cornwall. The festival of Golowan.

BEN: Festival of goblins?

ME: *Cackle, cackle!* Golowan. It's the Cornish word for midsummer. The celebrations begin on the twenty-third and end today. Ancient pagan customs are revived, like lighting fires and processions with torches. I'd like to be in Penzance today. The town is decorated with greenery and there's parties for children. It's become a major arts and cultural festival now – I'd love to go one day.

BEN: You could have a party in the garden with the fairies and garden gnomes. I'll get some colourful fairy cakes and you could have ice cream and jelly. Or I'll get some of those mini-trifles.

ME: Lovely!

* * * * * * * *

2.00 p.m. I'm sitting on the garden bench, afternoon sunbeams softly relaxing my soul, and enjoying a well earned rest from doing a spot of dusting in the sitting room. Ben sits beside me, bringing fairy refreshments, for a well earned rest after doing the Saturday shopping.

2.01 p.m. We celebrate what I now call The Goblin Festival, by gobbling trifle and fairy cakes.

2.07 p.m. I'm away with the fairies (high on sugar), watching my fairy wire sculpture (hanging from the bird table) twirl round, her copper hair and wings sparkling in the sunshine. Ben sends a message on his Smart-phone – I don't think it's to fairyland.

2.08 p.m.

ME: Do you know where I'd *really love* to go this summer?

BEN: *More than* visiting a dismal black lighthouse in a desolate looking marshland location, wearing your lighthouse hoodie?

ME: Not more, *the same as*.......... Well, this would mean more travelling and wearing fairy finery – although you don't have to.

BEN: Is there another festival of pixies, goblins and fairy folk coming up soon?

ME: I expect there is somewhere. But I'd like to visit Trentham Gardens in Staffordshire, to see Robin Dwight's huge fairy sculptures. It's a long journey, but I was thinking maybe we could stay at a B&B halfway? I'm hoping the gardens are still open to the public. Could you check on the internet for me?

BEN: Yep (replying to a message on his Smartphone).

ME: I've just read a beautiful fairy poem by Jean Ingalow. I'll read you the first verse.

> *Pray, where are all the little bluebells gone,*
> *That lately blossomed in the wood?*
> *Why, the fairies have taken each one,*
> *And put it on for a hood.*

BEN: Very nice dear.

ME: There's a poem entitled *Goblin Market* too.

> *Backward up the mossy glen*
> *Turn'd and troop'd the goblin men*
> *With their shrilled repeated cry –*

BEN: I must fly, I must fly (leaping to his feet).

ME: Meeting Alex for a coffee?

BEN: Yep. Enjoy your day with the pixies and fairies dear.

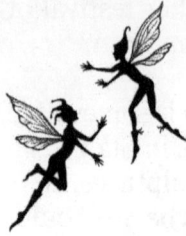

Sunday 29th

1.20 p.m.   I sit and peacefully sigh.

1.21 p.m.   Under a soft lilac blue sky.

1.22 p.m.   The busy bees buzz by.

1.23 p.m.   Fairies in fairyland fly.

1.24 p.m.   Ben sits beside me and asks –

BEN: *Why...* is there an empty milk carton in the washing machine?

ME: Another one for the absent-mind list!

WE LAUGH

ME: Listen to this.

BEN: Must I?

ME: It's sweet. By an unknown writer.

            Believe in the fairies
            Who make dreams come true.
            Believe in wonder,

The stars and the moon.
Believe in magic,
From fairies above.
They dance on the flowers,
And sing songs of love.
And if you just believe,
And always stay true,
The fairies will be there,
To watch over you!

BEN: Delightful.

ME: Do you remember this? (pointing to a calendar on my lap).

BEN: No.

ME: You gave it to me a few years ago for Christmas.

BEN: Did I?

ME: I love all the fairy paintings. I've been meaning to put two or three of my favourite ones in clip frames. I'm just enjoying another look. February is a lovely one – The Elfin Piper by Rene Cloke. April too – The Enchanted Glade by Daphne Constance Allen. Do you like them?

BEN: Very nice. Why are you giggling?

ME: I can't help noticing that in all the paintings by women, the fairies are wearing clothes. And in *all* the paintings by men, the fairies are naked. Look. Titania by John Simmons.

BEN: Tit – ania.

ME: And The Lily Fairy by Louis Ricardo Falero...... And Midsummer Night by John Atkinson Grimshaw.

BEN: Lovely (nodding with approval at the fairies with no clothes on). I expect the artists enjoyed showing off their life painting skills.

ME: Yes dear.

WE LAUGH

BEN: I see you've been doing some dusting, hope you've not been overdoing it.

ME: I've been pacing myself. Gradually getting the bathroom, sitting room and bedroom clean. Going to get my life dusted and nicer to live with too. Will make a formal complaint about the insulting surgeon, and change my doctor's surgery to your one.

BEN: My surgery is nearer home, and it always amuses you that it's opposite our vet.

ME: I've a good feeling about seeing the rheumatologist. Got my broomsticks crossed next to the fence.

BEN: Looks like a bird has done a big pooh down one of them.

ME: That's good luck!

WE LAUGH

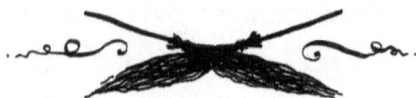

Monday 30th

12.10 p.m.   My Monday morning misty blues melted away. They became light pinks, pale lemons and lilacs (light and lovely as fairy cakes bought at a fairy festival), when I read a text message Ben had sent me during his lunch break.

I ASKED THE LION IN MY WARDROBE WHAT HE WAS DOING IN THERE – HE SAID IT WAS NARNIA BUSINESS

* * * * * * * *

12.35 p.m.   Watching *Loose Women* – 80% of the viewers do what I do!

12.36 p.m.   I laugh at myself. I have clothes in my wardrobe that I haven't worn for five, ten, fifteen (or more) years too, because they are too small for me – but one day I might fit into them again.

12.37 p.m.   The women on the *Loose Women* panel agree that this especially applied to jeans. I laugh again.

1.35 p.m.   I'm in the bathroom, sitting on the side of the bath, watching Cleopatra, who is standing on my weighing scales, staring at the dial. She should be on that programme, *Cats Make You Laugh Out Loud*.

* * * * * * * *

2.20 p.m.   I stand at the kitchen window, sipping minty tea, watching two large white butterflies dancing together. Three baby squirrels are prancing through the branches of the sycamore trees. I want to be dancing and prancing to fairy music with fairy folk, at a fabulous fairy festival again.

2.30 p.m.   As my fingers leisurely waltz through the pages of TV Weekly, I notice *Shrek 2* is on this week. I'll look forward to that. I so love the character, Donkey.

2.31 p.m.   I want to travel to the land of Far Far Away with Shrek.

2.32 p.m.   Or climb into my wardrobe and find myself in the land of Narnia.

2.33 p.m.   Or be rubbing shoulders (I mean fairy wings) with other fairy loving folk, at a fairy festival.

* * * * * * * * *

6.22 p.m.

ME: I had a funny moment with Cleo and Purrdi today.

Ben: That's nice.

ME: Lots of funny moments really.

BEN: Even better.

ME: I was lying on the sofa, Cleo and Purrdi fast asleep on my tummy and chest, watching one of my fave vintage sit-coms.

BEN: *Just Good Friends? Butterflies? Bread?*

ME: That reminds me, I must put bread on the shopping list. Can you get that nice one with seedy bits in again, it was really tasty.

BEN: Yes dear.

ME: Especially when it's toasted.

BEN: Yeah.

ME: Where was I?

BEN: On the sofa watching –

ME: *The Good Life*. The one where Barbara talks to her plants, to encourage them to grow.

BEN: Like you.

ME: Tom was jealous because she never talks to him with such a loving and endearing voice, which made me giggle – though I was trying not to, because I didn't want to disturb our hairy girls.

BEN: And that made you giggle more.

ME: They gave me cross little cat stares and twitchy tails. I felt guilty but couldn't help giggling again. That was a bad idea. They both plodded off to the kitchen on perturbed little paws, with *we-deserve-a-treat* cat body language. And y*ou-disturbed-our-beautiful-cat-dreams-so-give-us-a-Dreamies-treat* tail movements. *Or-as-you-seem-to-have-the-energy-to-giggle-so-much-maybe-you-could-plod-to-the-kitchen-to-open-a-fresh-can-of-tuna* intense cat stares and wild whiskers. So Dreamies and fresh tuna it was.

BEN: What a fun life you have.

ME: It's not a bad life. A *good life*. On a good day.

* * * * * * * *

7.45 p.m.

ME: I feel the need to be away with the fairies again, soon.

BEN: We could go to that country pub we went to after the dentist, it's surrounded by woodland. I'll drop you by a wood near the pub, and you can wander around in a floaty frock, till you find a fairy ring to stand in and make a wish – or have a little sing and dance, whatever takes your fancy. I'll have a pint in the pub, and a drink waiting for you after your adventure.

ME: Sounds good! The journey to the pub is enchanting. I love the way the trees make a cathedral-like canopy over the lane. And on a sunny day the tree leaves glow like cathedral stained glass windows, many shades of green. Then in autumn, golds and crimsons. Heavenly!

BEN: Yes dear, and you could do some tree hugging too.

ME: I know! Wanda of Weekly Witch, says hugging a tree reminds you that your roots go deep, and radiant healing strength grows within you. Each tree in a wood has an individual spirit, just as we have a unique energy. And you can find your inner power through meditating with a tree.

BEN: Wonderful.

ME: It is. Wanda says you can find strength after weathering a storm, because your roots grow deepest when the wind is strongest.

BEN: Do you feel a poem coming on?

ME: About heavenly cathedral trees, their slim branches the longest? The roots growing deeper when winds are the strongest?...... No, not today.

BEN: Oh, by the way. I got a reply from the marketing manager at Trentham Gardens, Amanda Dawson.

ME: What did she say?

BEN: It was a sweet e-mail, saying they have fifteen sculptures at the gardens. And just today, another fairy had flown in for the summer. They hope to welcome us soon.

ME: That's fabulous (huge smile).We could go when you have your next break at the end of August, it will be a lovely way to end the summer. We must book a cattery for our hairy girls (stroking Purrdita and Cleopatra to the tips of their tails). I do love a furry-tail ending. Don't you?

THE END

Dear Reader,

In case you are wondering, Verity got to see a very pleasant rheumatologist, and is coping well with the arthritis. Ben made an official complaint about the surgeon on her behalf and got a 'sort of' apology – better than nothing. And she has now registered at a new doctors surgery, where she has been treated well. And well treated.

Love Maria

PS   Thank you so much for reading my books.
     I hope you enjoyed them!

PPS Verity is looking forward to seeing the fairy sculptures at Trentham Gardens. So am I.